The Lungs in a Mechanical Ventilator Environment

Guest Editors

MEREDITH MEALER, RN, MS, CCRN
SUZANNE C. LAREAU, RN, MS, FAAN

CRITICAL CARE NURSING CLINICS OF NORTH AMERICA

www.ccnursing.theclinics.com

Consulting Editor
JANET FOSTER, PhD, APRN, CNS, CCRN

September 2012 • Volume 24 • Number 3

SAUNDERS an imprint of ELSEVIER, Inc.

W.B. SAUNDERS COMPANY
A Division of Elsevier Inc.

Elsevier Inc., 1600 John F. Kennedy Blvd., Suite 1800, Philadelphia, PA 19103-2899

http://www.theclinics.com

CRITICAL CARE NURSING CLINICS OF NORTH AMERICA Volume 24, Number 3
September 2012 ISSN 0899-5885, ISBN-13: 978-1-4557-3848-9

Editor: Katie Hartner
Developmental Editor: Donald Mumford

Critical Care Nursing Clinics of North America (ISSN 0899-5885) is published quarterly by Elsevier Inc., 360 Park Avenue South, New York, NY 10010-1710. Months of issue are March, June, September, and December. Business and Editorial Offices: 1600 John F. Kennedy Blvd., Suite 1800, Philadelphia, PA 19103-2899. Periodicals postage paid at New York, NY and additional mailing offices. Subscription prices are $144.00 per year for US individuals, $296.00 per year for US institutions, $76.00 per year for US students and residents, $192.00 per year for Canadian individuals, $371.00 per year for Canadian institutions, $219.00 per year for international individuals, $371.00 per year for international institutions and $111.00 per year for Canadian and foreign students/residents. To receive student/resident rate, orders must be accompanied by name of affiliated institution, data of term, and the *signature* of program/ residency coordinator on institution letterhead. Orders will be billed at individual rate until proof of status is received. Foreign air speed delivery is included in all *Clinics* subscription prices. All prices are subject to change without notice. **POSTMASTER:** Send address changes to *Critical Care Nursing Clinics of North America*, Elsevier Health Sciences Division, Subscription Customer Service, 3251 Riverport Lane, Maryland Heights, MO 63043. **Customer Service: 1-800-654-2452 (US and Canada); 314-447-8871 (outside US and Canada). Fax: 314-447-8029. E-mail: JournalsCustomerService-usa@elsevier.com (for print support) and JournalsOnlineSupport-usa@elsevier.com (for online support).**

Reprints. For copies of 100 or more of articles in this publication, please contact the Commercial Reprints Department, Elsevier Inc., 360 Park Avenue South, New York, New York, 10010-1710; Tel.: (212) 633-3813, Fax: (212) 462-1935, and E-mail: reprints@elsevier.com.

Critical Care Nursing Clinics of North America is covered in *MEDLINE/PubMed (Index Medicus)*, *International Nursing Index*, *Nursing Citation Index, Cumulative Index to Nursing and Allied Health Literature*, and *RNdex Top 100*.

Printed and bound by CPI Group (UK) Ltd, Croydon, CR0 4YY

Transferred to Digital Print 2012

Contributors

CONSULTING EDITOR

JANET FOSTER, PhD, APRN, CNS, CCRN
Texas Woman's University, College of Nursing, Houston, Texas

GUEST EDITORS

MEREDITH MEALER, RN, MS, CCRN
Research Instructor of Medicine, Division of Pulmonary Sciences and Critical Care Medicine, University of Colorado Denver School of Medicine, Aurora, Colorado

SUZANNE C. LAREAU, RN, MS, FAAN
Senior Instructor, College of Nursing, University of Colorado Denver, Aurora, Colorado

AUTHORS

ALEXANDER B. BENSON, MD
Assistant Professor of Medicine, Division of Pulmonary Sciences and Critical Care Medicine, University of Colorado Denver, Aurora, Colorado

SHANNON JOHNSON BORTOLOTTO, RN, MS, CCNS
Clinical Nurse Specialist, Critical Care, University of Colorado Hospital, Aurora, Colorado

SUZANNE M. BURNS, MSN, RRT, ACNP, CCRN, FAAN, FCCM, FAANP
Professor Emeritus, University of Virginia School of Nursing, Charlottesville, Virginia

DEBAPRIYA DATTA, MD, FCCP
Division of Pulmonary, Critical Care and Sleep Medicine, University of Connecticut Health Center, Farmington, Connecticut

RONALD E. DECHERT, DPH, MS, RRT, FAARC
Department of Respiratory Care, University of Michigan Health System, Ann Arbor, Michigan

VALERIE A. ELLIOTT, MSN, ACNP
Acute Care Nurse Practitioner, Weinberg Intensive Care Unit, Johns Hopkins Hospital, Baltimore, Maryland

CARL F. HAAS, MLS, RRT, FAARC
Department of Respiratory Care, University of Michigan Health System, Ann Arbor, Michigan

CYNTHIA B. KARDOS, BSN, RN, BA
Critical Care Research Coordinator, Critical Care Research Department, Baystate Medical Center, Springfield, Massachusetts

JULIE N. KING, RN, MS, ACNP
Acute Care Nurse Practitioner, Weinberg Intensive Care Unit, Johns Hopkins Hospital, Baltimore, Maryland

SUZANNE C. LAREAU, RN, MS, FAAN
Senior Instructor, College of Nursing, University of Colorado Denver, Aurora, Colorado

MARY BETH FLYNN MAKIC, RN, PhD, CNS, CCNS, CCRN
Research Nurse Scientist, Critical Care, University of Colorado Hospital; Assistant Professor Adjoint, University of Colorado, College of Nursing, Anschutz Medical Campus, Aurora, Colorado

PAULA MCCAULEY, DNP APRN ACNP-BC
Interim Associate Dean, Associate Clinical Professor, University of Connecticut School of Nursing, Storrs; Critical Care, Surgery Division, University of Connecticut Health Center, Farmington, Connecticut

BARBARA A. MCLEAN, MN, RN, CCRN, CCNS, NP-BC, FCCM
Clinical Nurse Specialist, Nurse Intensivist, Division of Critical Care, Grady Memorial Hospital, Emory University, Atlanta, Georgia

MEREDITH MEALER, RN, MS, CCRN
Research Instructor of Medicine, Division of Pulmonary Sciences and Critical Care Medicine, University of Colorado Denver School of Medicine, Aurora, Colorado

MARILYN NIELSEN, RN-BC, MS
Manager, Clinical Informatics, Littleton Adventist Hospital, Centura Health System, Littleton, Colorado

WASEEM OSTWANI, MD
Department of Pediatric Critical Care Medicine, University of Michigan Health System, Ann Arbor, Michigan

AMY J. PAWLIK, PT, DPT, CCS
Senior Physical Therapist, Therapy Services, University of Chicago Medical Center; Program Coordinator, Cardiac and Pulmonary Rehabilitation, University of Chicago Medical Center, Chicago, Illinois

JODI SARACINO, RN-BC, BSN
Clinical Informatics, Catholic Health Initiatives, Englewood, Colorada

SUSAN S. SCOTT, MSN, RN, CCRN
Unit Educator for Medical and Surgical Intensive Care Unit, Baystate Medical Center, Springfield, Massachusetts

Contents

Pulmonary critical care nurses have played a prominent role in the ICUs from the inception of critical care units. This article describes how the history of pulmonary critical care nursing has evolved and discusses a few of the challenges in the years to come: stress imposed by working in a critical care environment, enhancing the care of patients by altering patterns of sedation and promoting early mobilization, and dealing with increasing infection rates.

Critical patients presenting with acute respiratory failure (ARF) offer a plentiful, dynamic, and complex picture, which requires a deep understanding of gas exchange, pulmonary dynamics, and mechanical ventilation strategies. The most frequent cause of ARF is chronic disease with exacerbation. Interventions treating acute exacerbation, along with ventilatory support, physical therapy, and evidence-based strategies, may improve immediate outcomes. However, follow-up is essential and for the chronic obstructive pulmonary disease patient the goal is to avoid relapse or rehospitalization. This article discusses the evaluation of gas exchange failures, pulmonary mechanics, and the properties of obstructive airway disease as they relate to ARF.

Acute lung injury/acute respiratory distress syndrome (ALI/ARDS) continues to be a major cause of mortality in adult and pediatric critical care medicine. This article discusses the pulmonary sequelae associated with ALI and ARDS, the support of ARDS with mechanical ventilation, available adjunctive therapies, and experimental therapies currently being tested. It is hoped that further understanding of the fundamental biology, improved identification of the patient's inflammatory state, and application of therapies directed at multiple sites of action may ultimately prove beneficial for patients suffering from ALI/ARDS.

Three transfusion complications are responsible for the majority of the morbidity and mortality in hospitalized patients. This article discusses the respiratory complications associated with these pathophysiologic processes, including definitions, diagnosis, mechanism, incidence, risk factors, clinical management, and strategies for prevention. It also explores how different patient populations and different blood components differentially affect the risk of these deadly transfusion complications. Lastly, the article discusses how health care providers can risk stratify individual patients or patient populations to determine whether a given transfusion is more likely to benefit or harm the patient based on the transfusion indication, risk, and expected result.

Chronic obstructive pulmonary disease (COPD) is characterized by expiratory airflow limitation that is not fully reversible. Acute exacerbations in patients with moderate to severe COPD can cause severe hypoxia and persistent or severe respiratory acidosis, resulting in respiratory failure and the need for ventilator support. Acute respiratory failure, altered mental status, and hemodynamic instability associated with acute exacerbations of COPD are commonly encountered and require careful management in the intensive care unit (ICU). Noninvasive and invasive ventilator support in conjunction with pharmacotherapy can be lifesaving, although mortality remains high. It is important also to consider pulmonary rehabilitation and palliative care.

Pneumonia affects millions of people every year in the United States. Hospital-acquired pneumonia is associated with a mortality rate as high as 50%. Pneumonia is classified according to where it was acquired or by the infecting organism. This article explores the similarities and differences in three types of pneumonia seen routinely in the intensive care unit: community-acquired pneumonia, ventilator-associated pneumonia, and health care-associated pneumonia.

Approaches to mechanical ventilation (MV) are consistently changing and the level of ventilator sophistication provides opportunities to improve pulmonary support for critically ill patients. Advanced MV modes are used in the treatment of patients with complex pulmonary conditions. To achieve optimal patient outcomes MV modes that best meet the needs of patient's evolving pulmonary conditions are necessary. It's essential for nurses to integrate pulmonary MV knowledge in the care of critically ill patients. The purpose of this article is to describe the evidence supporting lung protective modes of MV used in the care of critically ill adults.

Weaning patients from long-term mechanical ventilation (LTMV) has been an important focus of clinical process improvement initiatives and research for decades. The purpose of this article is to describe the science that drives our current weaning practices, including (1) pre-weaning assessment, (2) individualized weaning plans, (3) weaning prediction, (4) the use of protocols and guidelines for weaning trials and sedation management, (5) timing of tracheostomy placement, and (6) system initiatives for the management of LTMV patients. Finally, this article discusses potential interventions for improving the outcomes of patients who require prolonged mechanical ventilation.

The purpose of this article is to provide an appreciation for a significant risk to quality of care affecting patients receiving mechanical ventilation: unplanned extubation. A summary of the current literature provides evidence-based recommendations for how to minimize this potentially dangerous complication. In addition, recommendations for proceeding after unplanned extubation are made.

Patients undergoing critical illness and mechanical ventilation are at risk of developing neuromuscular and neurocognitive impairments that can impact physical function and quality of life. Mobilizing patients early in the course of critical illness may improve outcomes. Recent literature on early mobilization is reviewed, suggestions for implementation are discussed, and areas for future research are identified.

It is estimated if each hospital implemented intensivist physician staffing, approximately 55,000 lives and $4.3 billion dollars could be saved in the United States. However, there is a limited supply of new critical care specialists as teaching hospitals have decreased the size of critical care programs for financial reasons. Tele-ICU can be used to provide coverage in facilities that cannot support a full-time specialist in critical care medicine and as an adjunct to facilities without 24-hour intensivist coverage. This article discusses the benefits and challenges of tele-ICU and its implications for nursing practice.

CRITICAL CARE NURSING CLINICS

Preface

Pulmonary Processes and Mechanical Ventilation in the ICU Patient

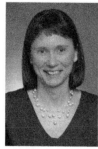 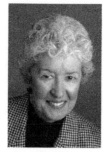

Meredith Mealer, RN, MS, CCRN   Suzanne C. Lareau, RN, MS
Guest Editors

The management of adult patients in the critical care environment is often complex and dynamic in nature. There have been rapid advances in life-sustaining technology in addition to new standard-of-care treatment for chronic and acute pulmonary disease processes. Despite these advances, mortality rates in critically ill patients with acute respiratory failure or acute exacerbations of chronic obstructive pulmonary disease remain high at 40% to 65%.[1] Improving patient outcomes requires a balance between advancements in the field of pulmonary science and adherence to evidence-based best practices.

This issue of *Critical Care Nursing Clinics of North America* addresses the challenges faced by critical care clinicians caring for patients requiring mechanical ventilation with or without underlying pulmonary disease. The issue begins with an introduction (Lareau and Mealer) to the history of pulmonary disease management in the intensive care unit (ICU) and future goals related to improving patient outcomes and improving the psychological health of nurses exposed to a stressful work environment.

The next five articles focus on the management of the most common pulmonary issues faced by the clinician in the ICU. McLean discusses the physiology, mechanics, and the evaluation of gas exchange failures as they relate to acute respiratory failure. Dechert, Haas, and Ostwani address the current scientific knowledge related to acute lung injury (ALI) and acute respiratory distress syndrome (ARDS). They discuss the pulmonary sequalae involved with ALI and ARDS, mechanical ventilation support, and adjunctive as well as experimental therapies to consider when caring for these patients. Pulmonary complications from the transfusion of blood products are addressed by Benson and include an overview of the terrible T's: transfusion-related

Crit Care Nurs Clin N Am 24 (2012) xi–xii
http://dx.doi.org/10.1016/j.ccell.2012.06.009
0899-5885/12/$ – see front matter

acute lung injury (TRALI), transfusion-associated circulatory overload (TACO), and transfusion-related Immunomodulation (TRIM). McCauley and Datta provide a summary of chronic obstructive pulmonary disease to include the clinical features, management of exacerbations, and pharmacologic and ventilator support of patients in the ICU. Finally, in the article by Scott and Kardos, pneumonia is discussed including community, health care, and ventilator-acquired pneumonias.

Mechanical ventilation strategies are discussed in the next three articles. The evidence supporting lung protective modes of mechanical ventilation in critically ill patients is presented by Makic and Bortolotto. Burns describes the current science related to mechanical ventilation weaning practices and includes preweaning assessments, individualized weaning plans, and protocols for weaning trials. Additionally, she discusses the timing of tracheostomy tube placement and interventions for improving outcomes in patients requiring prolonged mechanical ventilation. Last, Elliott and King describe the serious complication of unplanned extubation, which includes evidence-based recommendations to minimize this risk and interventions for proceeding after unplanned extubations.

The final two articles discuss relatively new innovations/interventions in the ICU. The first is an article by Pawlik describing the use of early mobilization in critical illness. The author provides evidence to support the benefit of early mobilization in preventing common negative sequalae of critical illness and discusses the continued efforts to determine the safety and outcomes of physical therapy in the critically ill patient population. Nielsen and Saracino discuss the fascinating topic of telemedicine as it relates to critical illness. They provide recommendations to implement telemedicine, summarize a tele-ICU care model, and describe the benefits and challenges involved with the adoption of this innovative practice.

In closing, we would like to thank all of the individual authors who contributed to this issue. We would also like to thank Dr Jan Foster, consulting editor for *Critical Care Nursing Clinics of North America*, for the opportunity to serve as guest editors.

Meredith Mealer, RN, MS, CCRN
Division of Pulmonary Sciences
and Critical Care Medicine
University of Colorado Denver
School of Medicine
12700 East 19th Avenue C272
Aurora, CO 80045, USA

Suzanne C. Lareau, RN, MS
College of Nursing
University of Colorado Denver
Education 2 North
13120 East 19th Avenue, Room 4327
PO Box 6511/C288-04
Aurora, CO 80045, USA

E-mail addresses:
Meredith.Mealer@ucdenver.edu (M. Mealer)
Suzanne.Lareau@ucdenver.edu (S.C. Lareau)

REFERENCE

1. Vincent JL, Mendonca A, Sprung C, et al. The epidemiology of acute respiratory failure in critically ill patients. Chest 2002;121(5):1602–9.

History of Pulmonary Critical Care Nursing and Where We Are Going

Suzanne C. Lareau, RN, MS[a], Meredith Mealer, RN, MS, CCRN[b],*

KEYWORDS

- Critical care • Intensive care nurses • Intensive care unit • Pulmonary • Nursing

KEY POINTS

- Pulmonary critical care nurses have played a prominent role in intensive care units (ICUs) from the inception of critical care units.
- The future calls for the protection of the emotional health of critical care nurses and addressing the burden of ICUs on patients by finding new ways to reduce infection and provide the kind of care needed for a healthier discharge from the ICU.

INTRODUCTION

Pulmonary diseases have been the stimulus behind the evolution of pulmonary and critical care nursing. Beginning with the care of tuberculosis (TB) patients in the 1800s, nurses are now providing highly skilled care for a variety of conditions, including the complex needs of patients with severe sepsis, acute lung injury (ALI), and/or acute respiratory distress syndrome (ARDS) and multiorgan system failure. The value of specialty nurses in the care of patients in the critical care setting has solidified. This article describes how the history of pulmonary critical care nursing has evolved and discusses a few of the challenges in the years to come.

CLINICAL HISTORY OF PULMONARY CRITICAL CARE NURSING

One cannot speak of pulmonary nursing without recognizing the longstanding contributions of nurses in the late 1800s who cared for TB patients in their homes, that is, the public health and visiting nurses. These nurses laid the foundation for specialty nurses, by providing care and comfort and orchestrating the myriad social needs of

Meredith Mealer received financial support from NIH grant no. K24 HL-089223.
The authors have nothing further to disclose.
[a] College of Nursing, University of Colorado Denver, Education 2 North, 13120 East 19th Avenue, Room 4327, PO Box 6511/C288-04, Aurora, CO 80045, USA; [b] Division of Pulmonary Sciences and Critical Care Medicine, University of Colorado Denver School of Medicine, 12700 East 19th Avenue C272, Aurora, CO 80045, USA
* Corresponding author.
E-mail address: Meredith.Mealer@UCDenver.edu

the patients (adults and children) to recover from life-threatening illnesses. In fact, early in the history of pulmonary nursing in the American Thoracic Society (ATS), it was nurses working with TB patients who were reporting (with usually a physician as the primary investigator) findings from their studies of TB, including directly observed therapy (DOT). DOT has become the model today for the successful treatment of TB. During the 1970s, pulmonary nurses in ATS were at the forefront of independently studying suctioning techniques and methods to reduce trauma to the airway.

In the 1950s during the polio epidemic, nurses continued to show their skills in both the technical and nursing management of patients in iron lungs (negative pressure ventilators). From there, it can be said, critical care nursing evolved rapidly. This evolution was coupled with the increase in knowledge and technology in caring for the cardiac patient. In the late 1960s, critical care nurses became a formidable voice. The American Association of Critical-Care Nurses (AACN) was formed and membership increased from 600 in the 1970s to a current membership of more than 88,000. AACN is now the premier organization to offer educational opportunities and networking for the estimated 500,000 nurses working in critical care settings.[1]

EDUCATION OF PULMONARY CRITICAL CARE NURSES

The educational preparation of pulmonary critical care nurses parallels that of all nurses. Initially, diploma preparation was the highest level of education of many critical care nurses. Quickly, baccalaureate degrees were more accessible, followed by the availability of master's programs directed at critical care nurses. With the exception of many public health nurses (an area that often required certification in public health), the only skills required to practice in a critical care setting were a desire to work in what at the time was considered a fast-paced setting and good clinical judgment and observation skills. This is not to say that the bedside nurse in the acute setting did not require these skills as well, as many critically ill patients are often in non–intensive care unit (non-ICU) settings. The level of knowledge and skill in delivering care to patients is more complex than ever before, in all areas of health care.

If pulmonary nursing was a predecessor of critical care nursing, then the National Association for the Study & Prevention of Tuberculosis (NTBRDA) was a key figure in advancing the education of these nurses. In 1944, the NTBRDA (later becoming the American Lung Association [ALA]) provided grants to the National Organization for Public Health Nursing and National League for Nursing (NLN) to advance the education of public health nurses in the care of TB patients. More than 20 years later, the NTBRDA awarded its first of many grants to the University of California San Francisco in 1968, to prepare pulmonary clinical nurse specialists (CNSs). Between 1974 and 1984, more than 12 universities were funded by the NTBRDA/ALA to prepare pulmonary CNSs.[2]

The 1970s also saw the beginning of educating critical care nurses in academic settings. Critical care CNS programs were offered by increasingly more institutions. For those not desiring to obtain formal training in an academic setting, but wishing to remain current in critical care, AACN offered education and training through its National Teaching Institute (National Teaching Institute & Critical Care Exposition®). By the mid-1970s, AACN began offering certification for critical care nurses. AACN certification in critical care nursing is not a requirement to work in most critical care units; however, many employers consider it evidence of major achievement as a critical care nurse.

FUTURE CHALLENGES

There are many important challenges facing the critical care nurse. One of the challenges for ICU nurses will be to deal with stress imposed by working in a critical care environment. Another challenge relates to enhancing the care of patients by altering patterns of sedation and promoting early mobilization. These have the potential for enabling patients to be discharged earlier from the ICU with a greater ability for independence. The ICU, like many areas of the hospital, is dealing with increasing infection rates. ICU nurses can play an integral role in reducing infection. The following section addresses nursing stress, provisions for early mobility, and infection.

The Psychological Health of Critical Care Nurses and Its Implications for the Nursing Shortage

A critical nursing shortage exists in the U.S. health care system, particularly in specialty areas such as the ICU, with reported turnover rates of 26%.[3] The nursing shortage is projected to grow to 260,000 registered nurses by 2025.[4] The reasons for this national crisis are multifactorial, yet one important component is the voluntary turnover of nurses due to dissatisfaction and stress related to the work environment. It has been reported that there is an increased prevalence of posttraumatic stress disorder (PTSD), secondary traumatic stress (STS), and burnout syndrome (BOS) among ICU nurses compared to general medical/surgical nurses.[5] The reasons for this are related to organizational factors as well as the cumulative effects of stress from repeatedly being exposed to the ICU work environment. ICU nurses delivering direct patient care have described the emotional stress, anxiety, and depression experienced from the daily confrontations with high patient mortality and morbidity and the ethical dilemmas that result from addressing end-of-life issues, prolonging life by artificial support, performing cardiopulmonary resuscitation, and participating in postmortem care. Recently, Mealer and colleagues[6] have been exploring the concept of resilience in critical care nurses and have reported that ICU nurses are significantly less likely to develop PTSD or burnout syndrome compared to ICU nurses who are not highly resilient (PTSD 25% vs 8%; BOS 85% vs 61%). Importantly, there are psychological characteristics of resilience that can be learned through cognitive-behavioral therapy, which include optimism, cognitive flexibility, developing a personal moral compass or set of spiritual beliefs, altruism, finding a resilient role-model or mentor, learning to be adept a facing fear, developing active coping skills and a supportive social network, exercising, and having a sense of humor. Mealer and colleagues[7] have conducted national qualitative interviews with highly resilient nurses and found that there are specific characteristics of resilience that have enabled these nurses to work in this tension-charged atmosphere for a long period of time while being able to maintain a healthy psychological profile. This has paved the way for the development of specific resilient target strategies that will potentially help prevent PTSD and BOS, thus ameliorating the ICU nursing shortage.

Daily Interruptions of Sedation and Early Mobilization of Critically Ill Patients on Mechanical Ventilation

The management of patients requiring mechanical ventilation has made advancements in recent years, which has improved outcomes and mortality rates. However, as patients survive critical illness, complications from prolonged hospital stays and immobilization have been associated with the financial burden of rehabilitation, and in some cases, major disability. A recent study conducted by

Schweickert and colleagues[8] determined that daily interruption in sedation combined with early mobilization of mechanically intubated patients, through physical therapy, improved the return of functional status at hospital discharge. In addition, these patients had a shorter duration of ICU-related delirium and the procedures were safe and well tolerated. Studies are underway to determine whether early mobilization in the ICU promotes successful discharge to home, reduces the burden of rehabilitative care after discharge, and improves long-term outcomes in these patients.

INCORPORATING EVIDENCE-BASED PRACTICE TO IMPROVE PATIENT OUTCOMES

The Institute of Medicine (IOM) issued a report in 2001, *Crossing the Quality Chasm: A New Health System for the 21st Century*,[9] that highlighted the gap between evidence-based practice and the quality of care in the United States. Despite this report and efforts by consumer groups, professional societies, and health care institutions to incorporate guidelines for the delivery of evidence-based care, there remains difficulty in the successful implementation of evidence-based practice. Two priorities in the ICU are preventing central line–associated bloodstream infections and incorporating severe sepsis bundles or standard order sets.

The U.S. Centers for Disease Control and Prevention (CDC) estimates that there are 800,000 preventable health care–acquired infections and 250,000 (30%) are acquired from central line bloodstream infections.[10] These infections cause an estimated 30,000 to 62,000 patient deaths annually. Johns Hopkins University championed a program addressing this issue, which resulted in a 66% reduction in central line bloodstream infections.[11] The program is a multidisciplinary effort between physicians and nurses, and includes three main processes: the Comprehensive Unit-Based Safety Program (CUSP); a model for Translating Evidence into Practice (TRiP); and a system to measure, report, and improve outcomes. This program and adapted versions of this program are being incorporated in ICUs nationwide, which hopefully will reduce the unacceptably high rate of preventable infections and deaths resulting from hospital-acquired infections.

Severe sepsis is a cascade of events caused by the body's systemic response to an infection, which results in single-organ or multiple-organ dysfunctions. The mortality rate associated with severe sepsis remains high. As a result, there has been an international effort aimed at awareness and improving patient outcomes. An international group of experts, spearheaded by the European Society of Intensive Care Medicine (ESICM), International Sepsis Forum (ISF), and the International Society of Critical Care Medicine (SCCM) developed the Surviving Sepsis Campaign (SSC). The purpose of the SSC is to provide evidence-based, multidisciplinary guidelines for the management and treatment of this syndrome. Included in the guidelines are education and training, screening tools for severe sepsis, fluid resuscitation guidelines, blood culture policy, and antibiotic use. This innovative campaign has resulted in improved resource utilization and improved quality of care to patients with sepsis.

The future of critical care nursing will be driven by the increasing demands that are currently being experienced in practice due to managed care and the increased acuity of patients being admitted to the ICU. The education of nurses must focus on developing highly specialized skills to manage new treatment methods and technologies. Finally, continued research efforts are needed to strengthen the discipline and improve patient outcomes.

SUMMARY

Pulmonary critical care nurses have played a prominent role in the ICU from the inception of critical care units. Close to half a million nurses work in a critical are setting. Opportunities for making an impact on patient care by keeping current with the latest in clinical care is in evidence by the thousands of nurses who attend the National Teaching Institute & Critical Care Exposition annually, while thousands of nurses in the United States and internationally have presented their research on various aspects of critical care. The future calls for the protection of the emotional health of critical care nurses and addressing the burden of ICUs on patients by finding new ways to reduce infection and provide the kind of care needed for a healthier discharge from the ICU.

REFERENCES

1. History of American Association of Critical-Care Nurses (AACN). Available at: http://www.aacn.org/wd/pressroom/content/historyofaacn.pcms?menu=aboutus. Accessed June 17, 2011.
2. Lareau S, Breslin E, Hansen M, et al. History of the American Thoracic Society assembly on nursing 1944 to 1998. New York: American Lung Association; 1998. Available at: http://www.thoracic.org/assemblies/nur/history/ala-support-of-nurses.php. Accessed June 17, 2011.
3. Stechmiller JK. The nursing shortage in acute and critical care settings. AACN Clin Issues 2002;13:577–84.
4. Buerhaus, PI, Auerbach DI, Staiger DO. The recent surge in nurse employment: causes and implications. Health Affairs 2009;28:657–68.
5. Mealer M, Burnham E, Goode C, et al. The prevalence and impact of post traumatic stress disorder and burnout syndrome in nurses. Depress Anxiety 2009;26:1118–26.
6. Mealer ML, Rothbaum B, Moss M. Highly resilient ICU nurses are less likely to develop psychological symptoms and disorders: results of a national survey [abstract]. Am J Respir Crit Care Med 2010;181:A2414.
7. Mealer M, Jones J, Moss M. Psychological characteristics of highly resilient ICU nurses: results of a qualitative study [abstract]. Am J Respir Crit Care Med 2011;183:A4114.
8. Schweickert W, Pohlman M, Pohlman A, et al. Early physical and occupational therapy in mechanical ventilated, critically ill patients: a randomized controlled trial. Lancet 2009;373:1874–82.
9. Institute of Medicine. Crossing the quality chasm: a new health system for the 21st century. Washington, DC: National Academies Press; 2001.
10. Consumers Union. To err is human—to delay is deadly. Consumers Report: Health. Younkers (NY): Consumers Union; 2009.
11. Pronovost PJ, Berenholtz SM, Goeschel C, et al. Improving patient safety in Michigan intensive care units. J Crit Care 2008;23:207–21.

Acute Respiratory Failure and Intensive Measures

Barbara A. McLean, MN, RN, CCRN, CCNS, NP-BC, FCCM*

KEYWORDS

- Oxygenation • Ventilation • Failure • Dynamics • Air trapping

KEY POINTS

- Critical patients presenting with acute respiratory failure (ARF) offer a plentiful, dynamic, and complex picture, which requires a deep understanding of gas exchange, pulmonary dynamics, and mechanical ventilation strategies.
- The most common cause of ARF is exacerbation of chronic obstructive disease and acute restrictive disorders, such as ARDS.
- Intervention designed to treat acute exacerbation (specific to chronic obstructive) along with appropriate and specific ventilatory support, physical therapy, and evidence-based intensive care unit strategies may improve the immediate outcomes for these patients.

INTRODUCTION

Impending or established respiratory failure is a common reason for admission of patients to the intensive care unit (ICU). The application of an artificial airway and mechanical ventilation support does not mean the patient has acute respiratory failure (ARF), as many patients in the ICU require airway support but only for short times. Acute respiratory failure is defined as a sudden deterioration of the ability to maintain alveolar–blood gas exchange. When confronted with a patient in ARF, the first priority is to identify and treat redeemable causes. Examples include a pneumothorax requiring a chest tube, acute pulmonary edema requiring diuresis, or an acute asthma exacerbation that may respond to bronchodilator therapy. In the absence of a readily reversible cause, most patients with ARF require mechanical ventilation, compelling a more involved ventilatory stay. Maintaining adequate arterial oxygenation while protecting the functional lung is the goal of highest priority in both traditional and more recent approaches to pulmonary management. The second goal is to determine and treat the underlying pathophysiologic condition whenever possible. The purpose

The author has nothing to disclose.
Division of Critical Care, Grady Memorial Hospital, Emory University, 80 Jesse Hill Jr. Drive SE, Atlanta, GA 30303, USA
* 1444 Cornell Road, Atlanta, GA 30306.
E-mail address: bmclean1@gmh.edu; bamclean@mindspring.com

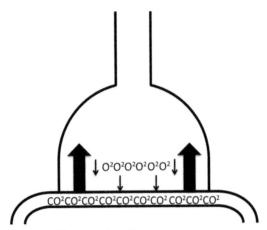

Fig. 1. Normal alveolar to capillary relationships.

of this article is to discuss the evaluation of gas exchange failures, pulmonary mechanics, and the properties of obstructive airway disease as they relate to ARF. More detailed and specific discussions of these and other particular states are included in other chapters.

PHYSIOLOGY

The primary goal of the pulmonary system is to promote an appropriate and reasonable gas exchange at the alveolar–capillary surface, generally evaluated at the bedside via pulse oximetry, measurement of arterial blood gases, and end-tidal CO_2 monitoring. Pulmonary function may be simply classified into ventilation and oxygenation, with ventilation and oxygenation further quantified by the ability of the respiratory system to eliminate CO_2 and form oxyhemoglobin. Although multiple factors (such as percent of atmospheric pressure that is oxygenated: F_iO_2) affect this gas exchange, the most basic properties involve alveolar recruitment and recoil, a narrow distance between each alveoli, and its dedicated capillaries and effective blood flow past the alveoli (**Fig. 1**). With this understanding of the basic physiology, it becomes clear that the measures of gas exchange are of the utmost importance in evaluating lung function.

EVALUATING AND DIAGNOSING GAS EXCHANGE FAILURES

As stated previously, ARF is the inability to maintain alveolar–blood gas exchange, resulting in a failure to remove CO_2 (due to hypoventilation) and/or failure to promote appropriate and proportionate O_2 uptake at the alveolar–capillary interface. One can evaluate the amount of O_2 added into the blood from the pulmonary circulation and the amount of CO_2 being removed from the blood in the pulmonary circulation by evaluating (via arterial blood gases) the amount of dissolved (P: pressure of) arterial O_2 as well as dissolved (P: pressure of) arterial and exhaled CO_2 (end-tidal CO_2).

Respiratory distress is the hallmark of ARF but hypoxemia may first present as an alteration in mental status or significant tachycardia. Hypercarbia may present in the same way. Typically the cutoff values for ARF are PaO_2 below 60 mm Hg and $PaCO_2$ above 50 mm Hg while breathing room air (contextual atmospheric pressure).

Table 1	
Differentiation of respiratory failure	
Type I Failure Acute Hypoxemic	**Type II Failure Acute Hypercapnic**
Pao_2 <60 mm Hg	$Paco_2$ >50 mm Hg
Patient at rest	Patient at rest
Breathing room air (F_Io_2 = 0.21 or 21% of the atmospheric pressure)	Breathing room air (F_Io_2 = 0.21 or 21% of the atmospheric pressure)

Oxygenation failure is typically labeled type I (hypoxemic), whereas type II (hypercapnic) is ventilation failure. A wide variety of disease states manifest respiratory failure of types II and I simultaneously (**Table 1**), creating a single or mixed respiratory failure. Although ARF is typically a mixed disorder, it may be helpful to consider these problems separately.

The goal of respiratory monitoring in any setting is to allow the clinician to ascertain the status of the patient's ventilation and oxygenation. The primary responsibility of the clinician is to identify and treat life-threatening conditions.

One of the simplest methods of evaluating patients and diagnosing or discussing their failure relates to the understanding of basic gas exchange.

CAUSES OF HYPOXEMIA

There are four primary problems that promote interference with the normal oxygenation of the arterial blood: hypoventilation, intrapulmonary shunt, diffusion impairment (altered diffusion distance), and ventilation perfusion mismatch ($\dot{V}/\dot{Q}$).

Hypoventilation

Although hypoxemia is not the most significant symptom of hypoventilation, it is a diagnostic factor. When minute ventilation (V_E) falls, $Paco_2$ will increase. In fact, so related is this property that if alveolar ventilation is halved, the $Paco_2$ will double. For hypoventilation to be the *cause* of hypoxemia, the arterial $Paco_2$ must be elevated (**Fig. 2**).

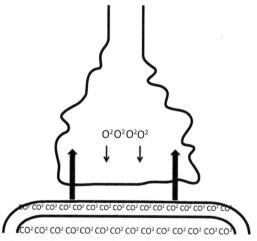

Fig. 2. Hypoventilated lung: alveoli to capillary relationships.

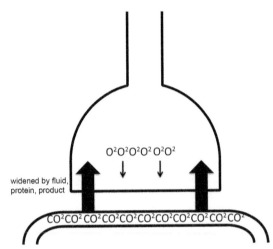

Fig. 3. Widened diffusion distance: alveoli to capillary relationships.

Clinical suspicion + high $Paco_2$ and low Pao_2. Responds to increase in V_E and/or high-flow oxygen.

Diffusion Distance

O_2 and CO_2 must cross the barrier created by the alveolar epithelium, the interstitial space and the capillary endothelium. That space between is typically fluid and product free, allowing gas to move rapidly across it. Diffusion is affected when an increase in anatomic distance and/or product (fluid, proteins, neutrophils) alters the ability of gas exchange between alveoli and capillary bed. Extravascular fluid is created when there is high pulmonary vascular pressure due to heart failure, loss of capillary barriers or high hydrostatic pressures, interferes with diffusion.

The gas in both directions must pass through the interstitial space that separates the alveoli and the capillary. Normally, equilibrium is achieved, that is, the PAo_2 will roughly equal the Pao_2. Whenever the interstitial space is widened, due to fluid or proteinaceous substance, oxygen exchange will decrease substantially. $Paco_2$ is generally unaffected in these disorders and the patient's Pao_2 is generally corrected by administering higher F_iO_2 to the patient (**Fig. 3**).

Clinical suspicion + low Pao_2 and normal $Paco_2$. Responds to high flow oxygen and F_iO_2.

Intrapulmonary Shunt

Right to left: Q_s/Q_T blood flow shunted/total blood flow
Proportionately low O_2 in the arterial blood or higher than expected CO_2 occurs when gas (alveoli) and blood (pulmonary capillaries) do not maximally exchange. Blood is allowed to pass from the right heart (mixed venous) to the left heart without being oxygenated. Whenever there is congenital dysfunction, profound consolidation, or dysfunctional alveoli that limit gas exchange, a shunt may occur. In addition, underventilated or unventilated alveoli also participate in the increase of shunt fraction. Shunt calculates the amount of blood passing from the right side of the heart through the pulmonary circulation and on to the left heart and then into the general circulation without receiving adequate oxygenation. This process commonly occurs

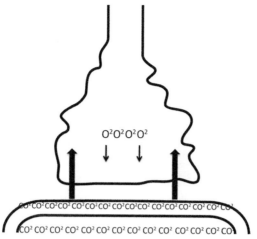

Fig. 4. Derecruited alveoli shunt: alveoli to capillary relationships.

when alveoli are not recruited on inspiration due to atelectasis, significant loss of the membrane integrity and surfactant, or the alveoli are flooded with fluid related to high pulmonary pressures and extravascular edema (**Fig. 4**).

A mathematical formula, based on both a mixed venous and systemic arterial blood gas, provides a calculation of intrapulmonary shunting. Normal physiologic shunt is 3% to 4% and may increase to 15% to 20% with acute respiratory distress syndrome (ARDS). The routine measurements of arterial blood gases (ABGs), chest radiograph, A-a gradient (A − a)DO_2, and PaO_2/F_iO_2 (P/F) ratio and the presence of refractory hypoxemia are more routinely used to support the assumption of shunt. Primary causes of intrapulmonary shunt are atelectasis and ARDS.

The greater the contribution from alveoli with mismatch (increasing shunt), the greater difference in or widening of the A-a gradient (A − a)DO_2 occurs. When the F_iO_2 is above 0.21, the A-a gradient (A − a)DO_2 becomes less accurate in the measurement of proportional gas exchange, although the difference should always be less than 150 mm Hg.

Clinical suspicion + low PaO_2 and normal $PaCO_2$. Does not respond to high flow oxygen and F_iO_2.

Alveolar Dead Space Ventilation

Alveolar dead space ventilation occurs when there are primary problems with pulmonary perfusion. Alveoli may be functional, compliant, and elastic, but in this condition the perfusion is proportionately lower than the ventilation. This is measured or evaluated as a high $\dot{V}/\dot{Q}$ mismatch, that is, ventilation is proportionately greater than perfusion. This is frequently seen with low cardiac output states, or pulmonary embolus (**Fig. 5**).

Clinical suspicion + low PaO_2 and normal to high $PaCO_2$. Does not respond to high flow oxygen and F_iO_2. The $ETCO_2$ gradient is wide as $PaCO_2$ is greater than $ETCO_2$.

Ventilation To Perfusion: $\dot{V}/\dot{Q}$ Mismatch

This general term refers to the relationship of gas distribution ($\dot{V}$) to the amount of blood ($\dot{Q}$), which passes the total alveolar surface in 1 minute. Normal alveolar

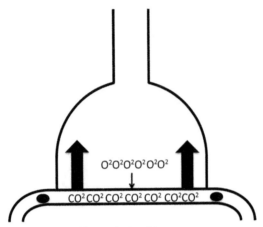

Fig. 5. Dead space: alveolar to capillary relationships.

ventilation occurs at a rate of 4 L/min, and normal pulmonary vascular blood flow occurs at a rate of 5 L/min. The normal $\dot{V}/\dot{Q}$ ratio is therefore 4 L/min divided by 5 L/min, or a ratio of 0.8, almost in a 1:1 ratio. Any disease process that interferes with either side of the equation upsets the physiologic balance, causing a $\dot{V}/\dot{Q}$ mismatch. This mechanism is the most common, frequently seen in the face of COPD as well as vascular disorders. Factors that may affect the $\dot{V}/\dot{Q}$ ratio include hypoventilation, COPD, oversedation, and both hyperdynamic and reduced cardiac output states. Conditions in which blood flow is inadequate for achieving gas exchange are known as increased dead space ventilation.

OXYGENATION MEASURES
A-a gradient (A − a)DO₂, also known as P(A − a)O₂/A − a DO₂

The A-a gradient $(A - a)DO_2$ or alveolar–arterial O_2 tension difference is a clinically useful calculation. The calculation is based on a model as though the lung were one large alveolus and the entire blood flow of the right heart passed around it (**Fig. 1**). Utilizing the rules of partial pressure as well as the laws of CO_2 production and CO_2 alveolar pressure, the theoretical alveolar PAO_2 is calculated (**Box 1**).

   Once the theoretical PAO_2 has been calculated, the gradient is achieved by subtracting the measured arterial PaO_2. The calculated "gradient" represents a mixture of blood circulated past alveoli presenting with ideal ventilation and the blood circulated past alveoli that have mismatch based on the physiology of dependent and

---

Box 1
Alveolar Po₂ (PAO₂) calculation

(F_iO_2) (barometric pressure water – vapor pressure) – $(PaCO_2/RQ)$ where the water vapor pressure (assumed) is 47 mm Hg and the RQ is assumed to be 0.8.

760 mm Hg – water vapor pressure (0.21) = 159 mm Hg

Measured $PaCO_2$ divided by RQ yields a proposed or assumed PAO_2.

Subtract the measured PaO_2 to find the A – a difference or gradient.

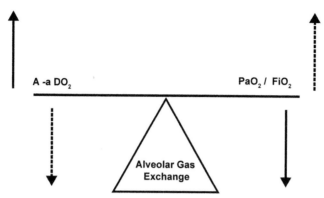

Fig. 6. Inverse relationship of gas exchange measures.

independent physiologic processes. In health, Pao_2 approaches PAO_2, so that the difference between the two, $P(A - a)o_2$, is small (<10 mm Hg in a young adult). Normal oxygenation requires that alveoli are functionally recruited, and appropriate blood flows past the alveoli to promote both oxygen uptake (alveoli–blood–hemoglobin) and CO_2 download (hemoglobin–blood–alveoli). Calculation of $P(A - a)o_2$ helps prevent the misinterpretation of lower blood oxygen as the major problem when patients present with CO_2 retention (as CO_2 displaces the oxygen).

PaO_2/F_iO_2 Ratio (P/F Ratio)

The Pao_2 divided by the F_iO_2 (Pao_2/F_iO_2 ratio or, more simply, P/F) can be used to more simply assess the severity of the gas exchange defect. The normal value for the Pao_2/F_iO_2 (F_iO_2 is expressed as a decimal ranging from 0.21 to 1.00) is 300 to 500. A value of less than 300 (>0.4 Fio_2) indicates gas exchange derangement, and a value below 200 (>0.4 Fio_2) is indicative of severe impairment and is one component utilized in the diagnosis of acute lung injury (ALI) and acute respiratory distress syndrome (ARDS).

The inverse relationships of the $A - a\ Do_2$ and the P/F ratio are important to consider when discussing the level of gas exchange failure (**Fig. 6**).

CARBON DIOXIDE MEASURES

CO_2 is one of the end products of tissue respiration. This byproduct is partially transported in the blood in a rapidly regulated, dissolved state as gas ($Paco_2$), ultimately affecting the blood pH. Most of the CO_2 in blood is present as bicarbonate ion, the amount of which ($Paco_2$) is determined by the ratio of carbon dioxide production ($\dot{V}co_2$) to carbon dioxide elimination as well as renal functional capabilities. CO_2 is more rapidly diffused than oxygen, requiring less functional alveolar gas exchange. For this reason, there must be significant dysfunction before CO_2 retention is noted. The metabolically produced CO_2, however, is mostly present as dissolved CO_2, added to the blood in the peripheral tissues and excreted by the lungs. In a steady state, the amount of CO_2 excreted through the lungs is exactly equal to the amount of CO_2 produced in peripheral tissues. Because the amount excreted is so easily influenced by minor changes in ventilation, the assurance of a steady state is particularly important. The amount of CO_2 excreted is primarily determined by the rate of alveolar ventilation [($\dot{V}_E$) minute ventilation: frequency (f)(V_E) exhaled tidal volume] as well as recoil of the alveoli and the time for exhalation.

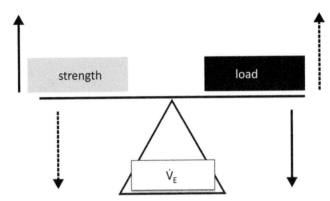

Fig. 7. Inverse Relationship respiratory strength and load.

Disorders that lower V_E may be understood by considering the relationship between respiratory muscle strength and respiratory system load. (**Fig. 7**). The neurologic–diaphragmatic–muscular function must affect enough negative intrathoracic pressure to overcome two major obstacles: the resistance to airflow in the conducting airways and the elastance (imposed resistance) of the lungs and chest wall and thoracic cage (which also includes the abdomen/diaphragm as the floor of the cage). In conditions in which the strength is poor or there is loss of any of the components, which maintain strength, V_E will decrease.

As long as the pressure generated is able to overcome these two mechanical loads, adequate alveolar ventilation will be sustained. If not, CO_2 accumulates as the alveoli may become overdistended with CO_2 rich gas. Assessment of neuromuscular function is important in patients with ARF, keeping in mind that it is the imbalance between strength and load that leads to hypercapnic respiratory failure. Successful treatment of acute hypercapnic respiratory failure requires restoration of the balance between the neuromuscular strength and respiratory system load.

Respiratory dysfunction involves inadequate gas exchange, ventilation, or both. Oxygenation requires matching pulmonary perfusion to alveolar recruitment, and CO_2 excretion relies primarily on ventilation. The strategy of ventilatory support may have a significant impact on outcome. Strategic ventilation is designed to achieve the goal of optimizing oxygenation uptake and CO_2 removal whenever possible. To provide the best possible strategy, one must understand the difference between obstructive and restrictive disorders (**Table 2**). A complete description is beyond the scope of this overview, but is addressed in the following chapters.

Because oxygenation occurs primarily during inspiration and the removal of CO_2 occurs during exhalation, the cyclical process must be appreciated. The purpose of mechanical ventilation is to support both cycles appropriately via combination of minute ventilation, FiO_2, inspiratory and expiratory time and mean airway pressures.

EPIDEMIOLOGY

The most common cause of ARF is the acute exacerbation of COPD, although restrictive disorders may present as ARF with little pre-existing disease.

COPD is generally considered a reventable and treatable disease hallmarked as primary airflow limitation. The airflow limitation is usually progressive and

Table 2
Differentiating obstructive and restrictive lung disorders

Obstructive Disease States, Impaired Exhalation, Impaired Minute Ventilation: CO₂ Retention:	Restrictive Disease States, Impaired Inspiration, Impaired Alveolar Recruitment: Hypoxemia, Refractory Hypoxemia
• COPD (emphysema, bronchitis, asthma, cystic fibrosis) • Neuromuscular defects (Guillian–Barré syndrome, myasthenia gravis, multiple sclerosis, muscular dystrophy, polio, brain/spinal injury) • Depression of respiratory control centers (drug-induced cerebral infarction, inappropriate use of high-dose oxygen therapy, drug/toxic agents)	• Pulmonary edema • ARDS • Anatomic loss of functioning lung tissue (pneumonectomy) • Restrictive pulmonary disease (interstitial fibrosis, pleural effusion, pneumothorax, kyphoscoliosis, obesity, diaphragmatic paralysis) • Pulmonary emboli • Atelectasis • Pneumonia • Bronchiolitis • Chest trauma (rib fractures) • Chest wall issues • Diffusion disturbances

associated with an abnormal inflammatory response of the lung to noxious particles or gases.[1]

To date, more than 52 million people have COPD, and the current estimation is that even though 12 million Americans have been diagnosed with COPD the same number of persons have the disease and have not been diagnosed.[2] COPD is the third leading cause of death in the United States. (For a more detailed discussion of COPD, please refer to COPD chapter).[3]

COPD is a clinical diagnosis that should be based on careful history taking, the presence of symptoms, and assessment of airway obstruction (also called airflow limitation) (see **Box 2**). Pulmonary function testing is the gold standard for an accurate and repeatable measurement of lung function and facilitates the diagnostic differential for asthma and COPD. COPD is also often misdiagnosed as asthma,[5] particularly in women; the diseases can be differentiated by postbronchodilator spirometry (significant improvement in exhaled volumes with asthma not COPD).[1] The standard diagnostic spirometry maneuver is a maximal forced exhalation (greatest effort possible) after a maximum deep inspiration (completely full lungs) (**Table 3**).

Box 2
Symptoms and assessment of COPD

Patients who present with:
• History of exposure to tobacco smoke, occupational dusts,
• cooking and biomass fuels
• Chronic cough, which may be daily and productive or intermittent and unproductive (sputum production: any pattern of sputum production may indicate COPD)
• Dyspnea on exertion, initially intermittent and becoming persistent
• Frequent exacerbations of bronchitis[1,3,4]

Table 3 Important spirometrics for COPD and asthma	
Measure	**Meaning**
FVC Forced vital capacity	The total volume of air that the patient can forcibly exhale in one breath.
FEV_1 Forced expiratory volume in 1 second	The volume of air that the patient is able to exhale in the first second of forced expiration.
FEV_1/FVC	The ratio of FEV_1 to FVC expressed as a fraction (previously this was expressed as a percentage of total volume ie, 0.7 means 70% of total volume) 0.7 and 0.8. Values <0.7 are a marker of airway obstruction, except in older adults, in whom values 0.65–0.7 may be normal.
FEV_6 Forced expiratory volume in 6 seconds	Approximates the FVC and in normal people the two values would be identical. Using FEV_6 instead of FVC may be helpful in patients with more severe airflow obstruction who make take up to 15 seconds to fully exhale.

PULMONARY MECHANICS

The basic properties of compliance and elastance are instrumental to the understanding of pulmonary dynamics (**Box 3**). This correlates back to the concept of strength and load, adding additional information for acute evaluation of the patient (**Fig. 7**). The compliant lung is one that is distendable, measured by the ability to achieve or receive a deep breath (vital capacity) with a small change in pressure. The evaluation of the pressure generated with a normal inspiration supports the evaluation of resistance to flow. The elastic lung is that which can recoil and exhale the deep breath with little to no air trapped inside (referred to as the functional residual capacity or volume of gas left in lung at end of a normal exhalation) (**Fig. 8**). The evaluation of the pressure generated with an inspiratory hold supports the evaluation of alveolar compliance.

A large amount of data can be obtained from patients who are mechanically ventilated: measurements of respiratory mechanics can be performed in dynamic a tidal volume breath: gas flows in or static (closure of exhalation valves immediately after a ventilated inspiration: gas is trapped in and does not flow out) conditions.

When patients are invasively ventilated, compliance and resistance can be recorded, while pressure, flow, and volumes are continuously monitored by the mechanical ventilator. Dynamic compliance is reflective of the overall resistance to the volume of gas delivered on a volume control breath and is measured as peak inspiratory pressure (PIP or P peak) (**Fig. 9**). Static compliance reflects the compliance

Box 3 Compliance and elastance of lungs

- Compliance is ability of lungs to stretch.
- Low compliance in fibrotic lungs (and other restrictive lung diseases) and when not enough surfactant.
- Elasticity (= elastance) is ability to return to original shape.
- Low elasticity in case of emphysema due to destruction of elastic fibers.
- Normal lungs are both compliant AND elastic.

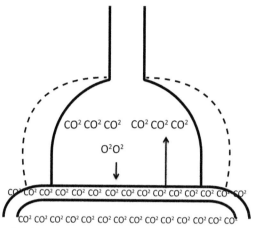

Fig. 8. Air trapping: alveoli to capillary relationships.

of the alveoli (the gas-exchanging surface) utilizing a ventilator induced inspiratory hold resulting in plateau pressure (P_{plat}) (**Fig. 9**).

Restrictive airway diseases generally present with significant loss of both dynamic and static compliance (increasing both pressures) as well as primary hypoxemia. An increase in peak inspiratory pressure without a concomitant increase in plateau pressure suggests an increase in airway resistance, while an increase in both peak inspiratory and plateau pressure suggests a decrease in the static compliance of the respiratory system (**Fig. 9**). Obstructive disorders are more likely to present with loss of recoil, profoundly significant air trapping (auto or intrinsic positive end-expiratory pressure [PEEP]) and a persistent and chronic hypercarbia (**Fig. 8**). Patients with COPD frequently have impaired oxygenation due to the loss of functional alveolar volume but have impaired ventilation related to increased dead space and poor respiratory mechanics. COPD patients with acute respiratory present providers with a critical challenge. Their respiratory systems are extremely fatigued, and they frequently lose their compensatory mechanisms (renal regulation, metabolic compensation). In addition, they may

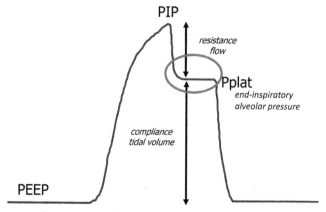

Fig. 9. The measured pressures and correlation to dynamics.

require mechanical assistance, but the ability to wean them effectively is of significant concern. Finally, although adjusting the minute ventilation to regulate the presence of $Paco_2$ seems to be a natural response, attention must be paid to time for exhalation and ventilatory support needs to be controlled to reduce air trapping as much as possible.[6]

PATHOPHYSIOLOGY
Failure To Exhale

Severe airflow obstruction associated with acute disease results in increasing residual volume and functional residual capacity, which may be referred to as dynamic hyperinflation or auto-PEEP in mechanically ventilated patients (**Fig. 8**).

The pathologic changes that occur in the lungs and give rise to the physiological abnormalities in COPD include mucus hypersecretion and ciliary dysfunction, airflow limitation and hyperinflation, gas exchange abnormalities, pulmonary hypertension, and eventually distal systemic effects. Patients with asthma present with very similar properties, evaluated by the process of air trapping, which is in the early stages airflow obstruction, is fully or partially reversible. As the disease progresses, the chronic airway inflammation creates edema, mucus, and eventually mucus plugging, which further decreases airflow, and increases air trapping. Eventually, irreversible changes in airway structure occur, including fibrosis, smooth muscle hypertrophy, mucus hypersecretion, injury to epithelial cells, and angiogenesis, further creating air trapping, a greater increase in functional residual capacity (air trapping or volume of gas that stays in the lungs after exhalation), and a decrease in forced vital capacity, eventually resulting in COPD (**Fig. 10**).

COPD comprises pathologic changes in four different compartments of the lungs (central airways, peripheral airways, lung parenchyma, and pulmonary vasculature), which are variably present in individuals with the disease.

At baseline, patients with COPD typically present with impaired ventilation (CO_2 removal) related to loss of recoil, increased dead space, and poor respiratory mechanics. Because of these baseline abnormalities, tolerance of acute pulmonary insults is poor and creates a significant exacerbation of the underlying process.

Patients with extreme dyspnea, altered mentation, or chest pain should go immediately to the emergency department.[4,5] Exacerbations (acute episodes) are a common cause of morbidity and mortality in COPD patients. Severe exacerbations are accompanied by a significant worsening of pulmonary gas exchange, mostly from increased ventilation–perfusion inequality and potentially by respiratory muscle fatigue. Worsening ventilation–perfusion relationships in exacerbations of COPD are multifactorial and relate to airway inflammation and edema, mucus hypersecretion, and bronchoconstriction (**Fig. 10**). These changes affect ventilation and cause hypoxic vasoconstriction of pulmonary arterioles, thus reducing perfusion, presenting with an increase in deadspace ventilation. Alveolar hypoventilation and respiratory muscle fatigue further contribute to hypoxemia, hypercarbia, and respiratory acidosis and may lead to severe respiratory failure and death. Hypoxia and respiratory acidosis produce pulmonary vasoconstriction, further decreasing perfusion and imposing an additional load on the right ventricle (RV). The pathogenesis of pulmonary hypertension in COPD is related to chronic hypoxia and hypercarbia with associated intravascular volume expansion.[7] If the ventricle compensates and the state is tolerated, RV hypertrophy may occur.[4] Reversible ischemic defects are also quite common (50%) in advanced COPD patients with left ventricular diastolic dysfunction without the presence of common risk factors and should be considered in the critical care evaluation.[8]

Patients with significant hypoxemia, cyanosis, edema, and/or arrhythmia should be admitted to the ICU for controlled oxygen treatment, ABG testing, and evaluation for pulmonary embolism (pulmonary embolism should be considered in all breathless

Normal Lungs and Lungs With COPD

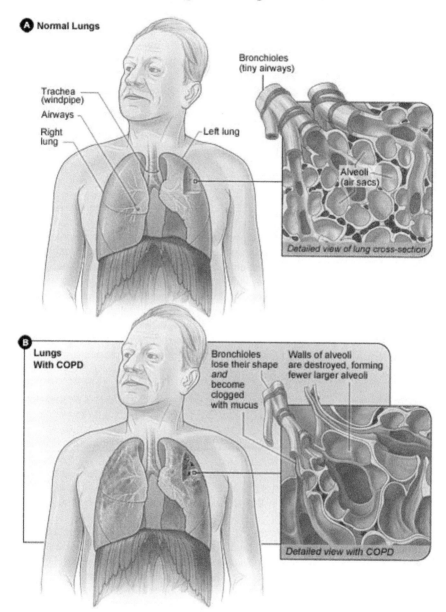

Fig. 10. Pathophysiology of COPD disorder. (*From* National Heart, Lung and Blood Institute. What is COPD? Available at: http://www.nhlbi.nih.gov/health/public/lungpublicdomainvisual.)

patients) or cor pulmonale.[1,4] The critical concepts of acute exacerbation encompass a wide constellation of problems, including deadspace ventilation, shunting, ventilation–perfusion mismatch, air trapping, right ventricular dysfunction, pneumonia, and systemic hypoxia. Early detection and intervention are vital.

Because of the deterioration of pulmonary structure and function, mechanical ventilation is often challenging in these patients. When mechanical ventilation of the COPD patient cannot be avoided, ventilator settings should aim at avoiding pulmonary hyperinflation and development of intrinsic PEEP (promoting air trapping and ineffective gas exchange). The use of noninvasive ventilation (NIV) is of particular interest in COPD patients, as it has been shown to be effective to avoid tracheal intubation during acute exacerbations.[6,9–11] Recent studies have introduced the inhalation of helium or nitric oxide as another method to treat these critical patients with significant reduction in mortality.[11,12] Early mobilization (walking) with transport ventilator and physical therapy also shows promise for the future. The effects on longer-term muscle strength, physical function, life quality, and resource utilization after hospital discharge of ICU patients are yet to achieve consensus, but may impact daily care in the ICU in the future.[13–15]

SUMMARY

Critical patients presenting with ARF offer a plentiful, dynamic, and complex picture, which requires a deep understanding of gas exchange, pulmonary dynamics, and mechanical ventilation strategies. The most frequent cause of ARF is chronic disease with exacerbation. Intervention designed to treat acute exacerbation (specific to COPD), along with appropriate and specific ventilatory support, physical therapy, and evidence-based ICU strategies, may improve the immediate outcomes for these patients. However, follow-up for any patient with ARF is essential, and for the COPD patient the goal of acute exacerbation treatment is to avoid relapse or rehospitalization, which affects approximately 30% of patients within 8 weeks after hospital discharge.[7] The goal of long-term management is to reduce risk of further exacerbations and interrupt or slow the progressive spiral of functional respiratory decline.

REFERENCES

1. Global Initiative for Chronic Obstructive Lung Disease (GOLD). Global strategy for the diagnosis, management and prevention of COPD. Available at: http://www.goldcopd.org/. Accessed June 1, 2012.
2. COPD: fact sheet. Available at: http://www.nhlbi.nih.gov/health/public/lung/other/copd_fact.htm. Accessed June 4, 2012.
3. Mannino D. COPD: epidemiology, prevalence, morbidity and mortality, and disease heterogeneity. Chest 2002;121:121s–6s.
4. Berry CE, Wise RA. Mortality in COPD: causes, risk factors, and prevention. COPD 2010;7:375–82.
5. Tinkelman DG, Price DB, Nordyke RJ, et al. Misdiagnosis of COPD and asthma in primary care patients 40 years of age and over. J Asthma 2006;43:75–80.
6. Ward NS, Dushay KM. Clinical concise review: mechanical ventilation of patients with chronic obstructive pulmonary disease. Crit Care Med 2008;36(5):1614–9.
7. Weitzenblum E. Chronic cor pulmonale. Heart 2003;89:225–30.
8. Bhattacharyya P, Acharjee D, Ray SN, et al. Left ventricular diastolic dysfunction in COPD may manifest myocardial ischemia. COPD 2012;9(3):305–9.
9. Donaldson GC, Wedzicha JA. COPD exacerbations: epidemiology. Thorax 2006;61:164–8.
10. Berry CE, Wise RA. Mortality in COPD: causes, risk factors, and prevention. COPD 2010;7:375–82.
11. Maggiore SM, Richard JM, Abroug F, et al. A multicenter, randomized trial of noninvasive ventilation with helium-oxygen mixture in exacerbations of chronic obstructive lung disease. Crit Care Med 2010;38:145–51.

12. Curtis JR, Cook DJ, Sinuff, T, et al; The Society of Critical Care Medicine Palliative Noninvasive Positive Pressure Ventilation Task Force. Noninvasive positive pressure ventilation in critical and palliative care settings: understanding the goals of therapy. Crit Care Med 2007;35(3):932–9.
13. Hopkins RO, Spuhler VJ, Thomsen GE. Transforming ICU culture to facilitate early mobility. Crit Care Clin 2007;23(1):81–96.
14. Bailey P, Thomsen GE, Spuhler VJ, et al. Early activity is feasible and safe in respiratory failure patients. Crit Care Med 2007;35(1):139–45.
15. Needham DM. Mobilizing patients in the intensive care unit: improving neuromuscular weakness and physical function. JAMA 2008;300(14):1685–90.

Current Knowledge of Acute Lung Injury and Acute Respiratory Distress Syndrome

Ronald E. Dechert, DPH, MS, RRT[a],*, Carl F. Haas, MLS, RRT[b],
Waseem Ostwani, MD[c]

KEYWORDS

- Acute lung injury • Acute respiratory distress syndrome • Molecular biology
- Cytokines • Molecular biology

KEY POINTS

- Acute lung injury/acute respiratory distress syndrome (ALI/ARDS) continues to be a major cause of mortality in adult and pediatric critical care medicine.
- Cytokines contribute to the pathophysiologic state via receptor-mediated signaling pathways that effect target cell responses.
- The application of molecular biology techniques into the field of critical care has both improved our understanding of this biological response and identified a number of potential therapeutic targets.

INTRODUCTION

The first published report describing the clinical syndrome currently referred to as acute respiratory distress syndrome (ARDS) occurred in 1967.[1] Since this landmark work by Ashbaugh and colleagues,[1] numerous investigators have reported clinical trials and observations of adult patients who exhibited the clinical sequelae associated with this syndrome with varying outcomes. Current evidence suggests that the mortality associated with this syndrome has been decreasing while substantial morbidity persists.[2–5]

Acute lung injury (ALI) and ARDS involve a heterogeneous process in the lungs that results in diffuse alveolar damage. The current characteristics associated with

[a] Department of Respiratory Care, University of Michigan Health System, 8-720 Mott Hospital, 1540 East Hospital Drive, SPC 4208, Ann Arbor, MI 48109, USA; [b] Department of Respiratory Care, University of Michigan Health System, UHB1H203, 1500 East Medical Center Drive, SPC 5024, Ann Arbor, MI 48109, USA; [c] Department of Pediatric Critical Care Medicine, University of Michigan Health System, 8-720 Mott Hospital, 1540 East Hospital Drive, SPC 4208, Ann Arbor, MI 48109, USA
* Corresponding author.
E-mail address: rdechert@umich.edu

Crit Care Nurs Clin N Am 24 (2012) 377–401
http://dx.doi.org/10.1016/j.ccell.2012.06.006
0899-5885/12/$ – see front matter © 2012 Published by Elsevier Inc.

ccnursing.theclinics.com

Table 1
Causative factors associated with ALI and ARDS

Direct Pulmonary Insult	Indirect Pulmonary Insult
• Pneumonia	• Sepsis
• Aspiration (especially gastric content)	• Blood transfusions
• Pulmonary contusion	• Nonthoracic trauma
• Fat emboli	• Reperfusion injury from cardiopulmonary bypass
• Near-drowning	• Acute pancreatitis
• Pneumonitis (oxygenation, smoke inhalation, radiation, bleomycin)	• Drug overdose

ALI include bilateral infiltrates on chest radiograph, Pao_2 to Fio_2 ratio less than 300, no evidence of left ventricular failure evidenced by a pulmonary artery occlusive pressure less than 18 mm Hg or central venous pressure less than 14 mm Hg, and need for invasive mechanical ventilator support. ARDS is a subset of patients whose Pao_2 to Fio_2 ratio is less than or equal to 200. ALI (or ARDS) is associated with a variety of causative factors, which can be grouped into two general categories: those associated with direct lung injury via the airways and those associated with indirect lung injury via the blood stream (**Table 1**).[6,7] More recently, investigators have focused on an extension of direct factors associated with iatrogenic lung injury induced by mechanical ventilation,[8–12] currently referred to as ventilatory induced lung injury (VILI). VILI can be further stratified as lung injury attributable to volume (volutrauma) or pressure (barotrauma). This article discusses the pulmonary sequelae associated with ALI and ARDS, the support of ARDS with mechanical ventilation, available adjunctive therapies, and experimental therapies currently being tested.

PULMONARY SEQUELAE ASSOCIATED WITH ARDS

Regardless of whether injury originates within or outside of the lung, the lung injury is associated with a systematic inflammatory response.

Early researchers developed a conceptual model of ARDS that involved three distinctive phases: (1) exudative or acute, (2) fibroproliferative, and (3) resolution. This basic model remains the hallmark for the physiologic changes associated with ALI and ARDS.

Exudative Phase

In this early presentation, the histology demonstrates marked diffuse alveolar damage, increased accumulation of neutrophils, vasodilation, endothelial cell damage, and pulmonary edema, secondary to increased vascular permeability[13–16] as shown in **Fig. 1**.

Analysis of bronchoalveolar lavage samples obtained from ARDS patients have identified numerous mediators present in this milieu, which include cytokines, oxygen radicals, activated complement, and leukotrienes (**Table 2**).[17,18] These histologic changes produce the characteristic symptoms associated with the exudative phase of ARDS. Physiologically, hypoxemia results from interstitial and alveolar flooding that contributes to intrapulmonary shunting and atelectasis.[19,20] The alveolar flooding also results in a decrease in pulmonary compliance.

The exudative phase of ARDS is believed to occur over 3 to 7 days from the onset of lung injury. From 33% to 50% of all deaths associated with ARDS occur during this early phase.[21]

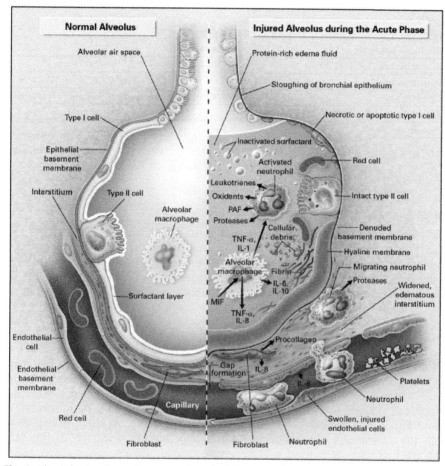

Fig. 1. Physiologic alternations associated with onset of ARDS. (*Reprinted from* Ware L, Matthay M. The acute respiratory distress syndrome. N Engl J Med 2000;342(18):1334–49; with permission.)

Fibroproliferative Phase

Persistent ARDS leads to increased alveolar and parenchymal damage, pulmonary hypertension, and pulmonary fibrosis. After a few days of lung injury, proliferation of alveolar cells, endothelial cells, and fibroblasts occurs. If ARDS persists during this proliferative phase, alveolar scarring (fibrosis) and multiple organ failure may occur. The development of pulmonary fibrosis and multiple organ failure contributes to mortality during the late phase of ARDS. During this phase, activated lung fibroblasts secrete a procollagen that is cleaved to create a type III collagen, referred to as Pro-Collagen Peptide-III (PCP-III). Clark and colleagues demonstrated in 1995 that the presence of PCP-III in the BAL fluid of ARDS patients is significantly correlated with mortality, and PCP-III appears to reflect the development of pulmonary fibrosis.[22] This finding was confirmed and further extended in subsequent investigation performed by Chesnutt and colleagues in 1997.[23]

Table 2 Proinflammatory mediators associated with the development of ARDS	
Mediator Category	Mediators
Tumor necrosis factors (TNF)	TNF-α, TNF-β
Interleukins (IL)	IL-1β, IL-2, IL-6, IL-10, IL-12
Chemokines	IL-8, growth-regulated peptides, MIP-1, MCP-1
Colony-stimulating factors (CSF)	G-CSF, GM-CSF
Interferon (IFN)	IFN-β

Abbreviations: MCP-1, Monocyte Chemotactic Protein-1; MIP-1, Macrophage Inflammatory Protein-1.

Resolution Phase

For those who survive the exudative and fibroproliferative phases of ARDS, the final phase results in either death or recovery. The most recent large-scale, multicenter trial identified the mortality of ALI/ARDS at approximately 35%.[24] Death in this population is commonly associated with the development of multisystem organ failure (MSOF). The sequencing of MSOF from the onset of ARDS has not been delineated, so the relative contribution to mortality for a given organ system remains unclear. This may be an area of important epidemiologic research for the future.

The successful resolution of ARDS may be related to some early changes in the histology of the alveoli.[25] Neutrophils make up the majority of the cellular component of BAL fluid in patients with ALI/ARDS. As the lung injury resolves, neutrophils are replaced by alveolar macrophages. It is believed that these macrophages, although capable of inducing further lung injury, play an important role in the resolution of the injury. **Fig. 2** demonstrates current understanding of the complex changes beginning with the proliferative processes and proceeding through resolution of the ALI. Important changes associated with this phase include epithelial repopulation, reabsorption of the alveolar fluid, clearing of the protein residue associated with the influx of the edema fluid observed in the exudative phase of lung injury, and finally resolution of fibrosis.[6,7,26,27]

The discovery of long-term effects on the pulmonary function of survivors associated with the onset and resolution of ALI has provided additional impetus to the systematic evaluation of quality-of-life (QOL) measures in this population. Previous investigators examined and reported the on QOL changes in survivors after hospital discharge.[26–31] McHugh was the first to conduct and report such a systematic investigation.[29] Similar to long-term changes in pulmonary function testing observed in ARDS survivors, there was a decrease in QOL immediately after extubation with a gradual improvement over time. The findings of abnormal QOL indices have been replicated by those of other researchers using a variety of instruments to measure QOL alterations.[30–32] Hopkins identified significant neuropsychological deficits after resolution of ARDS.[33] Davidson reported that ARDS patients had worse health-related QOL than the control groups.[28] More recently, several investigators reported on QOL changes that extended beyond the original 2 years postdischarge in survivors of ARDS. Dowdy and colleagues reported in a meta-analysis in 2006 involving 13 studies and 557 patients substantial reductions in all domain scores (using the SF-36) except mental health and role physical domains.[34] Similarly, Adhikari and colleagues reported in 2011 that depression

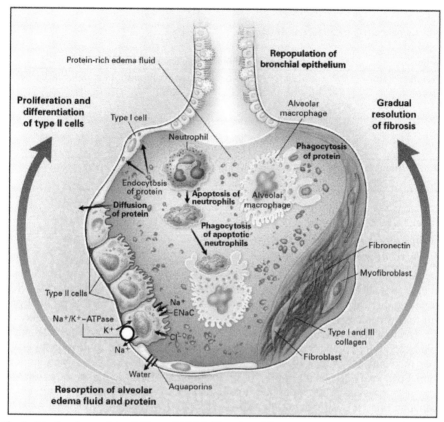

Fig. 2. Mechanisms of resolution of ARDS. (*Reprinted from* Ware L, Matthay M. The acute respiratory distress syndrome. N Engl J Med 2000;342(18):1334–49; with permission.)

symptoms and memory complaints persisted for up to 5 years after discharge in 64 survivors of ARDS.[35] These persistent findings of altered QOL after hospital discharge in ARDS survivors have prompted the ARDS-USA Foundation to request that physicians caring for ARDS patients should make them aware of short-term and long-term alterations following hospital discharge.[36] The health care burden has not been delineated but one would expect that as survivors increase, so will the burden on the health care providers.

Alveolar Mediators

A vast number of cellular mediators have been implicated in the pathogenesis of ARDS.[25,37–42] **Tables 2** and **3** list several mediators that have been associated with the development of ARDS. These mediators are believed to have an important role in the early inflammatory process through the recruitment and activation of neutrophils and mononuclear phagocytic cells. Of particular interest are various interleukins and tumor necrosis factor (TNF). Perhaps the most important of these are TNF-α, interleukin (IL)-1β, IL-8, and IL-10. **Table 3** briefly outlines the role each of these mediators play in the development and resolution of ARDS. Interventional therapies have targeted the roles these mediators play in mitigation of the inflammatory process associated with ARDS.

Table 3
Primary pulmonary mediators of ARDS

Action	Mediator	ARDS Phase	Pathophysiologic Response
Proinflammatory	TNF-α	Early	Fever, hypotension, impairment of endothelial barrier function.
	IL-1β		
	IL-8		Mediates neutrophil infiltration.
	MCP-1		Facilitates recruitment of monocytes into alveolar airspace.
Anti-Inflammatory	IL-10	Late	Downregulates cytokine production by macrophages.
	TGF-β		Deactivates monocytes.

MECHANICAL VENTILATORY SUPPORT
Ventilator-Induced Lung Injury

Mechanical ventilation is the main therapy supporting gas exchange and acid–base balance in patients with respiratory failure due to ARDS. Although considered a life-saving therapy, mechanical ventilation can also cause lung injury that pathophysiologically mimics ARDS, a condition referred to as ventilator-induced lung injury or VILI. The ventilator-associated complications of oxygen toxicity[43] and barotrauma[44] have been long appreciated in the development of VILI; however, only recently have other mechanisms of injury been identified and potentially of more clinical importance. Lung injury can occur at the two opposite ends of the breathing pattern: when regional lung tissue is overstretched during inspiration (volutrauma),[9,12,45] and when open lung units are repetitively allowed to collapse during expiration and re-expand on consecutive breaths (atelectrauma).[45] Both types of injury can cause inflammatory mediator release into the blood stream and trigger end-organ failure (biotrauma), which may increase mortality.[11,46–48] Limiting inspired volume and peak inspiratory pressure may be critical in minimizing volutrauma, while strategies that maintain patency of recruited lungs units, such as with positive end-expiratory pressure (PEEP), may be helpful in minimizing atelectrauma.

LUNG PROTECTIVE VENTILATION STRATEGIES
Low Tidal Volume and Pressure Limitation

The current standard of care for ventilatory management of patients with ALI/ARDS was described in a randomized controlled trial (RCT) by the NIH ARDS Network,[24] which demonstrated a 22% relative (9% absolute) mortality reduction. This study suggested that volutrauma was minimized when tidal volume (V_T) was targeted to 6 mL/kg of predicted body weight (PBW), and reduced to as low as 4 mL/kg PBW to maintain the end-inspiratory plateau pressure (P_{plat}) 30 cm H_2O or less. Although the initial study was conducted using volume control ventilation, the current recommendation allows pressure ventilation as long as V_T is monitored and limited.

When V_T is reduced to maintain target P_{plat}, set respiratory rate should be increased, up to a maximum of 35 breaths/min, in an attempt to maintain a pH of 7.30 to 7.45. Increasing the set rate reduces the available time for exhalation, so care must be taken to minimize the creation of auto-PEEP.[49] Administering a buffering agent might be necessary to maintain pH higher than 7.15 so V_T and P_{plat} can be kept within target, particularly when allowing permissive hypercapnia.

Table 4													
Fio$_2$/PEEP tables													
Lower PEEP/higher Fio$_2$ table													
Fio$_2$	0.30	0.40	0.40	0.50	0.50	0.60	0.70	0.70	0.70	0.80	0.90	0.90	0.90	1.00
PEEP	5	5	8	8	10	10	10	12	14	14	14	16	18	18–24
Higher PEEP/lower Fio$_2$ table													
Fio$_2$	0.30	0.40	0.40	0.50	0.50	0.60	0.70	0.70	0.70	0.80	0.90	0.90	0.90	1.00
PEEP	5	8	10	12	14	14	16	16	18	20	22	22	22	22–24

With the use of smaller volumes and faster rates, it is often perceived that patients may be uncomfortable and require more sedation than patients receiving larger V$_T$s, but this perception has not been borne out in clinical studies.[50] Interestingly, a recent study suggested that the use of a neuromuscular blocking agents (NMBAs) for the initial 48 hours of mechanical ventilation was associated with reduced mortality in patients with severe ARDS.[51] Although the trend in recent years is to reduce the use of NMBAs to minimize the incidence of prolonged muscle weakness, judicious short-term use early in the process may improve patient-ventilator synchrony and reduce VILI.[52]

PEEP and Recruitment Maneuvers

Oxygenation is supported by ventilator adjustments in both PEEP and Fio$_2$, to target a Pao$_2$ of 55 to 80 mm Hg or Spo$_2$ of 88% to 95%. PEEP is an anti-derecruitment pressure, helping to keep the airways and alveoli open that were inflated during the previous inspiration. By maintaining lung volumes at end-expiration, oxygenation is improved by reducing the ventilation–perfusion mismatch. It is generally accepted that a PEEP of less than 5 cm H$_2$O is harmful to patients with ARDS because it allows significant atelectrauma. Pressures of 8 to 15 cm H$_2$O are appropriate for most patients to minimize atelectrauma; however, higher levels may be required in patients demonstrating potential for lung recruitment.[53] How to determine the best level of PEEP to apply is controversial.

There are two basic strategies for setting the PEEP level: either using a table for all patients or individualizing the level by assessing a change in gas exchange or respiratory mechanics. The Fio$_2$/PEEP table concept was popularized by the ARDS-net studies, and many other RCTs have used this strategy in at least one arm of their study. Two Fio$_2$/PEEP tables have been described, one using a lower PEEP level than the other for a given Fio$_2$ (see **Table 4**). Both tables have been shown to be safe, but neither to be superior to the other.[54] It has been recommended that the low PEEP table be used in patients demonstrating a low potential for lung recruitment, while the higher PEEP table be used for patients demonstrating a higher degree of potentially recruitable lung tissue.[55]

An individualized approach to setting PEEP is encompassed in the Open Lung concept, which is summarized in the saying, "open the lung and keep it open."[56] This approach involves four steps: (1) opening the lung by increasing inflation pressure to a level above the critical opening pressure of a significant number of alveoli, (2) gradually reducing PEEP from a modestly high level (approximately 20–25 cm H$_2$O) until the critical closing pressure is reached indicating lung derecruitment, (3) reapplying the pressure used in step one to reopen collapsed lung units, and (4) applying a PEEP level slightly above that associated with the critical closing level.[57]

Other individualized approaches include obtaining information about respiratory mechanics from a pressure–volume loop during a slow inflation[58,59] and deflation[60,61] or via the pressure–time graphic scalar,[62,63] but both are influenced by increased abdominal and pleural pressure, not just lung pathology.[64] Measuring esophageal pressure to calculate the actual transpulmonary pressure (P_{tp}), or the pressure used to stretch the lung, is attractive. P_{tp} reflects the pressure difference between the pressure inside versus outside of the lung. In addition to setting PEEP in this manner,[65] calculating P_{tp} at end-inspiration may inform us when high plateau pressure is safe or harmful.[66-68]

Three large multicenter RCTs have compared lower levels of PEEP to higher levels of PEEP: the ARDSnet ALVEOLI study,[54] the Canadian/Australian LOVS trial,[69] and the French EXPRESS trial.[70] Each used high versus low PEEP strategy combined with a low-V_T strategy. The ARDSnet and Canadian studies used the same PEEP/Fio_2 table. The Canadian trial also allowed P_{plat} up to 40 cm H_2O and the application of intermittent increased inflation pressures (recruitment maneuvers) in the high-PEEP group. The French trial used a similar low-PEEP table, but individualized high-PEEP by increasing PEEP to attain a P_{plat} of 28 to 30 cm H_2O. None of these studies reported a mortality difference, and the ARDSnet and French studies were stopped early for futility. A meta-analysis by Briel and colleagues analyzed the data of the 2299 patients from these three trials.[71] For all patients, there was no difference in hospital mortality, although higher PEEP was associated with reduced intensive care unit (ICU) mortality, total rescue therapies (ie, inhaled nitric oxide [NO], prone positioning, high-frequency oscillatory ventilation, extracorporal membrane oxygenation), and death after rescue therapy. When stratified by the presence of ARDS or ALI at baseline, there was also a reduced hospital mortality (34.4% vs 39.1%) and more ventilator-free days at day 28 (12 vs 7 d) in the higher PEEP group for patients with ARDS at baseline. There was no difference in the incidence of barotrauma or use of vasopressors. Interestingly, there was a trend toward improved mortality in the lower PEEP group with ALI at baseline.

Recruitment maneuvers (RMs), as previously described, are part of the Open Lung concept, but they are also used as a stand-alone strategy to improve oxygenation. The ideal RM method has not been identified. A recent systematic review of recruitment maneuvers included 40 studies totaling almost 1200 patients.[72] The sustained inflation method (ie, continuous positive airway pressure [CPAP] of 35–50 cm H_2O for 20–40 seconds) was used most often (45%), followed by pressure control using high inspiratory pressure and PEEP settings (23%), incremental PEEP (20%), and a high V_T/sigh (10%). Oxygenation was significantly increased after a RM, but the duration of this effect was short lived. Adverse effects during the RM included hypotension (12%) and oxygen desaturation (8%), both of which were generally transient, returning to baseline shortly after the RM, and rarely caused the RM to be prematurely discontinued. Serious adverse events, such as barotrauma (1%) and arrhythmias (1%) were infrequent. The authors concluded that given the uncertain benefit of transient improvement in oxygenation, routine use of RMs could not be recommended or discouraged and they should be considered on an individualized basis in patients with a life-threatening hypoxemia.

It has been suggested that studies of recruitment maneuvers showing oxygenation improvement but short duration of benefit may not have set PEEP to an adequate level after the RM, and that those that showed no benefit used relatively low recruiting pressures or applied them late in the course of disease.[73] Iannuzzi demonstrated that the pressure control method (peak pressure of 45 cm H_2O with PEEP of 16 cm H_2O for 2 minutes) compared to the sustained inflation method (CPAP 45 cm H_2O for 40 seconds) improved oxygenation to a larger degree and was better tolerated hemodynamically.[74] A recent study of 50 ARDS patients evaluated the timing of lung recruitment and hemodynamic effects of a RM using a constant pressure of 40 cm H_2O for 40 seconds.[75] More than 98% of the volume ultimately recruited was attained within 10 seconds of applying the pressure. Mean and systolic blood pressures were stable for the first 10 seconds but became significantly reduced ($P<.01$) from baseline at 20 and 30 seconds. The authors recommended that when using the constant pressure RM method, the duration should be limited to 10 seconds to maximize recruitment and minimize hemodynamic compromise.

Current evidence suggests that that RMs should not be routinely used on all ARDS patients unless severe hypoxemia persists. RM might be used as a rescue maneuver to overcome severe hypoxemia, to open the lung when setting PEEP, or after evidence of acute lung derecruitment such as a ventilator circuit disconnect.[76]

Airway Pressure Release Ventilation

Airway pressure release ventilation (APRV) was originally described in 1987.[77,78] This mode of ventilation uses a breathing system that allows "unrestricted breathing" at two levels of CPAP. APRV is often described as "upside down IMV" in that intermittent mandatory ventilation allows spontaneous breathing at a low CPAP level that is intermittently raised to provide mechanical tidal inflation (ie, a mandatory breath). APRV encourages spontaneous breathing at a high CPAP level that is intermittently released to a lower CPAP level, allowing an increased exhaled volume to augment spontaneous minute ventilation.

There are two schools of thought on how to set the lower CPAP level and duration of release. One practice sets the low CPAP to 0 cm H_2O and a release time short enough to create air-trapping (auto-PEEP).[79] The other practice is to set the low CPAP to a more traditional PEEP level (eg, 10–15 cm H_2O) and the release time sufficient to allow complete exhalation before transition to the high CPAP level (ie, no auto-PEEP).[80] In both methods, a majority of the breathing cycle is at the high CPAP level (generally an I:E ratio of >4:1), resulting in a higher mean airway pressure (P_{mean}) compared to conventional pressure and volume ventilation modes. All potential spontaneous breathing occurs at the high CPAP level, as the release period is so short that it allows only exhaled volume and there is no time for spontaneous breathing.

Spontaneous breathing during APRV improves the ventilation–perfusion distribution in dependent lung regions, enhances venous return and improves cardiac output in the face of increased P_{mean}, and requires less sedation.[81] Although APRV-like settings can be applied to a passive patient, it is essentially pressure-control inverse-ratio ventilation if the patient is not spontaneously breathing.

Nonrandomized studies in ALI/ARDS patients report APRV to be associated with a lower peak inspiratory pressure,[82,83] less sedation and vasopressor use, improved oxygenation,[84,85] and possibly improved mortality.[85] Four RCTs of APRV have been reported. Multiple trauma patients at risk for ARDS were randomized to either APRV (n = 15) or pressure-control ventilation (PCV) (n = 15).[80] This study is often referenced in support of APRV, as it was associated with shorter duration of mechanical ventilation and ICU stay, as well as less use of vasopressors and inotropes. A significant limitation to this study, however, was that the control group was paralyzed for the first 72 hours, which may have given a bias toward the APRV group who were allowed to spontaneously breathe. A study of ARDS patients randomized to APRV (n = 30) or synchronized intermittent mandatory ventilation (SIMV) (n = 28) found lower inspiratory pressures were required in the APRV group but no difference was observed in gas exchange, hemodynamics, or ventilator-free days at day 28.[86] Computer-assisted tomography was performed on 37 ALI patients at baseline and 7 days after randomization to APRV or SIMV. It was found that the change in the amount of nonaerated lung tissue was similar ($P = .65$), suggesting that neither form of ventilation was superior.[87] In addition, in a study of trauma patients randomized to APRV (n = 31) or SIMV with pressure support ventilation (n = 32) found no difference in ventilator days, ICU days, incidence of pneumothoraces or ventilator-associated pneumonia, percent of patients requiring a tracheostomy, percent of patients failing the assigned modality, or mortality rate.[88]

APRV is available on all current generation ventilators and has become popular in many centers, although the evidence at this time does not support its routine use.

High-Frequency Oscillatory Ventilation

High-frequency oscillatory ventilation (HFOV) delivers very small V_Ts (0.1–3 mL/kg PBW) at rapid rates (180–900 cycles/min or 3–15 Hz).[89] Conceptually it applies high level CPAP with a wiggle. Oxygenation is supported by adjusting Fio_2 and P_{mean}, while ventilation in affected by increasing the drive pressure or reducing the rate of oscillation. Although counterintuitive, reducing the rate improves minute ventilation by allowing more time for the piston to move back and forth, generating a larger stroke or V_T.[90]

HFOV has been shown to aid in lung recruitment, improve oxygenation, and reduce histologic lung damage and inflammation in animals.[91–94] Adult clinical case series suggest that HFOV is safe and at least as effective as conventional ventilation, but has generally been applied as a rescue therapy for refractory hypoxemia.[95–103] Two RCTs compared HFOV to conventional ventilation in ARDS patients. In one study, 148 patients were randomized to HFOV (n = 75) or conventional ventilation (n = 73). They found early improvement in oxygenation with HFOV, but the difference was not sustained beyond 24 hours.[104] Although there were no differences in any other measured parameter, there was a trend ($P = .102$) toward improved mortality in the HFOV group (37% vs 52%). A limitation of this study was that the control group did not receive what is now considered a lung protective ventilation strategy. In an RCT of ARDS patients randomized to HFOV (n = 37) and conventional ventilation (n = 24), no difference was found in survival without supplemental oxygen or requiring ventilator support, mortality, therapy failure, or crossover to the other ventilatory strategy.[105] A post hoc analysis found a better treatment effect in patients with higher oxygenation requirement at baseline. Two RCTs of HFOV in conjunction with prone positioning in ARDS patients found that proning, regardless of ventilation method, improved oxygenation[106] and that HFOV maintained the oxygenation gained from the prone position better than conventional ventilation when returned to the supine position.[107]

HFOV theoretically should provide the optimal protective ventilation pattern with very small V_Ts to minimize volutrauma, and a high P_{mean} for recruitment to minimize atelectrauma. To provide the most lung protective settings, it is suggested to use a high oscillation pressure amplitude (starting at 90 cm H_2O) coupled with the fastest frequency tolerated (ideally >6 Hz) targeting a pH of 7.25 to 7.35.[100,108,109]

Two large RCTs are underway and the results are anticipated to be available in the next several years. Hopefully these studies will better inform us if HFOV results in better outcomes compared to conventional management, particularly if used earlier in the course of ARDS.

ADJUNCTIVE THERAPIES
Inhaled NO

In the lung, NO derives from several cellular sources, forming networks of paracrine (a form of cell signaling) communication. In pulmonary vessels, NO produced by endothelial cells is a powerful vasodilator. In the airways, NO originates from epithelial cells and from adventitial nerve endings to induce smooth muscle relaxation. Activated macrophages can also produce large quantities of NO during lung immunological reactions. In the normal pulmonary circulation, NO not only mediates vasodilation, but also opposes vasoconstriction, prevents platelet adhesion, controls growth of smooth muscle, and influences the composition of the extracellular matrix.

In patients with ALI/ARDS who are exposed to hypoxia; impaired endothelial NO production contributes to the increased vasomotor tone and vascular remodeling, leading to sustained pulmonary hypertension. Exogenous NO gas delivered via the airspaces is a selective pulmonary vasodilator in aerated portions of the lung, which cause blood flow to redistribute toward ventilated areas. This results in improved matching of perfusion to ventilation, and therefore arterial oxygenation, without causing concomitant systemic vasodilation.[110–116] The effect of NO on oxygenation and pulmonary artery pressure may allow more time for the lungs to recover.

Several randomized clinical trials enrolling adults with ARDS from various causes have failed to show a survival benefit for inhaled NO when compared to conventional mechanical ventilation alone[117–121] Approximately 60% of patients demonstrate improvement in oxygenation. A meta-analysis of 12 RCTs found no significant effect of NO on hospital mortality, duration of ventilation, or ventilator-free days. NO improved oxygenation until day 4. Patients receiving NO had an increased risk of developing renal dysfunction.[122]

Likewise, in children with severe hypoxemic respiratory failure, although NO at 20 parts per million (ppm) acutely improved oxygenation and lowered mean pulmonary artery pressure,[123] there was no clear effect on survival.[124] As 35% of children who initially did not respond to NO did so after lung volumes were increased by HFOV, combined use of HFOV and NO may provide more predictable improvement in children with ARDS.[125]

Adverse and potential toxic effects of inhaled NO are methemoglobinemia, increased nitrogen dioxide, peroxynitrite anion, platelet inhibition, increased left ventricular filling pressures, and rebound hypoxemia and pulmonary hypertension.[126,127] These side effects are seen mostly with high concentrations of inhaled NO (>20 ppm), prolonged usage, and high Fio_2.

Inhaled NO should be considered in patients with life-threatening hypoxemia that fail conventional interventions. Once NO is initiated, the amount of NO is titrated up until an improvement in oxygenation is observed. If there is no response after 30 minutes, then gradually discontinue its use. If there is a response, Fio_2 should be weaned to an acceptable level and then inhaled NO should be decreased to the lowest dose necessary to maintain the target oxygenation. Inhaled NO is not normally used for longer than 3 to 4 days.

Extracorporeal Life Support

Extracorporeal life support (ECLS) has been used for nearly 30 years as a "rescue" therapy for pediatric acute respiratory failure; however, optimal use relies on appropriate patient selection. ECLS is considered when patients are refractory to conventional therapies and have a potentially reversible lung injury.

ECLS for severe ALI/ARDS uses a veno–venous (VV) life-support circuit versus veno–arterial (VA). With ECLS, the circuit removes blood from the patient and circulates it through a membrane oxygenator to relieve the lungs from their main function of gas exchange and allow the lungs to heal.

Current Extracorporeal Life Support Organization (ELSO) registry data indicate that overall survival in this cohort remained relatively unchanged over the past 15 years at 57%, but this treatment is currently offered to increasingly medically complex patients. VA ECLS is the most common mode of support in pediatric respiratory failure patients, but a gradual increase of the usage of VV ECLS for this population has been witnessed especially with the advancement of ECLS technology and significantly lower odds of injury for VV compared to VA support.[128]

Clinical factors associated with mortality with ECLS include precannulation ventilator support longer than 2 weeks and lower precannulation blood pH.[128] The need to institute ECLS before the development of ventilator-induced lung injury was demonstrated by several early studies in pediatric[129,130] and adult[131] patients.

The OI is the oxygenation index, a measurement that characterizes oxygenation as a function of the intensity of ventilatory support (OI = $[100 \times P_{mean} \times FiO_2]/PaO_2$). A trend in the OI may be beneficial in assisting the clinician in identifying patients who may benefit from ECLS, before they transition into a syndrome of irreversible multiorgan dysfunction.[132,133]

The use of ECLS is associated with significant risks, mostly because of the need for anticoagulation and large indwelling vascular access. Commonly reported complications include clots in the circuit, hemorrhage at cannulation sites, and infection.[134–136]

ECLS should be performed as part of a protocol at experienced medical centers. ECLS is not usually considered for patients with contraindications to anticoagulation or for those who have been ventilated with high pressures for more than 1 to 2 weeks.[137]

EXPERIMENTAL THERAPIES
Modulating the Regulation of Lung Edema Clearance

An important component of maintaining homeostasis of lung function is the ability to continuously clear alveolar lining fluid. The most important factor that preserves the alveolar space from flooding is the resistance of the epithelial cells to injury. Even in the setting of endothelial barrier injury, preservation of epithelial function serves to keep extravasated fluid in the interstitium, where lymphatic drainage can accommodate an increased need for fluid removal, thus sparing the air space from edema formation. It has been observed that patients who have higher alveolar fluid clearance rates have improved survival than patients with a lower than normal alveolar fluid clearance rate.[138] Experimental settings of endothelial injury (eg, systemic endotoxemia) support that epithelial function in fluid clearance is dependent on β-adrenergic agonist stimulation of Na^+,K^+-ATPase-dependent sodium transport.[139]

A phase II trial of intravenous infusion of β-agonist in lung injury trial showed promising results with a reduction in extravascular lung water. However, a multicenter phase III study had to be stopped because of significant increase in mortality with the administration of β-agonists.[140–143] These findings were consistent with the acute lung injury ALTA trial of aerosolized β-agonist.[141,144]

$β_2$-agonists may have a direct effect on cardiovascular morbidity in patients with risk factors for cardiovascular disease.[145] Many patients with critical illness have comorbid cardiovascular disease. It is therefore possible that some patients experience adverse cardiovascular events, including occult cardiac ischemia during their critical illness.

Although together the results of these trials will likely answer the question concerning the use of β-agonists in the treatment of ALI in adults, questions remain about the role of β-agonists in the prevention of pulmonary edema and ALI. The majority of animal studies of ALI demonstrating a benefit used β-agonists as a preinjury treatment. After prolonged hypovolemic shock or high V_T ventilation, there is failure of β_2 adrenergic upregulation of alveolar fluid clearance,[146,147] and these models may more accurately reflect the clinical setting.

Recent human studies support this. The prophylactic use of β-agonists reduced the development of high-altitude pulmonary edema[148] and was found to reduce pulmonary edema and improved oxygenation in patients undergoing lung resection.[149] Other studies are ongoing to investigate this possibility. The Beta Agonist Lung Injury Trial (BALTI)—prevention is a trial of inhaled salmeterol as a prophylactic treatment given to patients undergoing elective transthoracic esphagectomy to prevent the development of acute lung injury.[150] The Beta-agonists for Oxygenation in Lung Donors (BOLD) is testing the effect of nebulized albuterol on oxygenation and lung transplantation rates in brain-dead organ donors.[151] When the outcomes of these trials are known, a more complete understanding of the indications for β-agonists in the management of pulmonary edema and ALI may become clear.

Future directions may consider application of gene therapy because preclinical studies have shown that overexpression of the α- and β-subunits of Na^+,K^+-ATPase can decrease lung edema formation in mouse models.[152]

Blocking Adhesion Molecules

The characteristic steps taken by leukocytes to extravasate from blood to the site of inflammation caused by either exogenous or endogenous stimuli have been recognized and summarized for about two decades as the "three-step" paradigm of inflammatory cell recruitment that involved rolling, activation, and adhesion. Extensive research in this field has resulted in the expansion of the three-step leukocyte adhesion cascade to include further adhesive processes between leukocytes and the endothelium, such as the slow rolling, the locomotion, or crawling as well as the transendothelial migration.[153–163] The interaction between the leukocytes and the endothelium comprises a variety of adhesive and migratory molecular events including low-affinity transient and reversible rolling adhesions, integrin-dependent firm adhesive interactions, and migratory events of the leukocytes through the endothelium and beyond that, such as the penetration of the basement membrane and migration in the interstitial space.[157,163]

As our understanding of the role of adhesion molecule expression has unfolded, the goal of anti-adhesion molecule therapy has become an intriguing pursuit. Numerous preclinical animal trials have demonstrated that anti-adhesion molecule antibodies, such as anti-ICAM-1,[164,165] anti-E-selectin,[166] anti-L-selectin,[167] and anti-P-selectin[165,168] were able to inhibit neutrophil accumulation in the lung and subsequent tissue injury. Despite these encouraging results, to date, no human trials have successfully used anti-adhesion molecule strategies.

It is important to recall that the leukocyte-adhesion molecule cascade is a highly conserved and adaptive host response necessary for pathogen clearance, as evidenced by individuals who suffer recurrent bouts of infection as a result of leukocyte adhesion deficiency (LAD) syndromes 1 and 2. The molecular basis of the defects associated with LAD-1 and LAD-2 are absent expression of the β-integrins (the counter-receptors for ICAM-1) and absence of sialyl-Lewis X (the carbohydrate ligand for selectins), respectively.[169,170] In light of these observations from **nature's** experiment, investigators must approach the strategy aimed at disrupting this cascade carefully, especially in the setting of an invading pathogen.

Targeting Cytokine Production

Although a number of cells produce cytokines, those of mononuclear-leukocyte lineage, such as the peripheral blood monocyte (in indirect lung injury) and the alveolar macrophage (in direct lung injury), appear to be principal sources. A number of agents have shown promise in **deactivating** these cells as a means of inhibiting cytokine production. Anti-inflammatory cytokines such as IL-10[171] and TGF-β[172] and other pharmacologic agents such as ketoconazole[173,174] and lisofylline[175] display potent monocyte deactivating properties and have been touted as potentially promising therapeutic strategies in ARDS, though this potential has not been realized in those studies performed to date.

Cytokine Neutralization

After their discovery, cytokines were considered as strictly proinflammatory molecules on the basis of their contribution to this pathophysiology of sepsis and ALI/ARDS. In addition, because of the proximal role cytokines play in the inflammatory cascade and their autocrine amplification effects, investigators have attempted to directly block their activity either by antibody neutralization (eg, anti-TNF-α antibody) or receptor blockade (eg, IL-1Ra). Although these strategies proved promising in preclinical trials, their ultimate clinical efficacy in human trials has been disappointing.[176,177] There are many reasons for this observation, including inaccurate modeling of the human disease, poor identification of underlying risk factors, and limitations on statistical power analysis.[178] Other factors weighing against the success of this strategy include the fact that cytokines are likely to be increased before the clinical presentation of a critically ill patient. In addition, the cytokine cascade has been discovered to be highly redundant and interlinked, making it unlikely that inhibition of any single mediator will prove beneficial in the context of the clinical trials that are limited by size. Finally, given the heterogeneity of both the triggering insults and the patients' comorbid conditions and immune response, it is unlikely that all patients with ALI/ARDS are battling uncontrolled proinflammation. It is likely that a subset of individuals exist in a relatively immunocompromised state as a result of overexpression of anti-inflammatory molecules rendering the patient at substantial risk for overwhelming infection as the cause of respiratory failure.

One notable exception to this approach has been the success observed with the use of the anti-TNF agent etanercept in idiopathic pneumonia syndrome (IPS) after bone marrow transplantation. When etanercept is applied early to patients with this form of acute, noninfectious lung injury, remarkable success has been achieved in decreasing radiologic evidence of lung edema and clinical resolution of ALI sufficient to warrant a phase II/III trial sponsored by the national Bone Marrow Transplant Trials Network and Children's Oncology Group.[179,180]

Blocking of Chemokines or Chemokine Receptors

Chemokines appear to play a central role in the activation and recruitment of neutrophils to the lung in ALI/ARDS, and as a result chemokines have become important therapeutic targets in many inflammatory states including ALI/ARDS. Monoclonal antibodies directed against IL-8 have been shown to decrease neutrophil influx and tissue injury in a number of animal models of lung injury[181–183] Because of these encouraging preclinical results, anti-IL-8 antibody has been considered for testing in human ARDS; however, it has come to light that antigen–antibody complex formation between IL-8 and anti-IL-8 may trigger an increased inflammatory response and has been associated with higher mortality.[184,185] Thus, whether this approach will continue to have merit is debated and instead, alternative approaches to attenuating the effects of chemokines have been suggested. Besides antibody neutralization, targeting the chemokine receptors has become a novel therapeutic target for clinical investigators.[186] As a result, it is possible that chemokines may be successfully inhibited in both a selective and effective manner in the near future.

Application of Genomics to ARDS

ARDS is a highly heterogeneous disease process with respect to both etiology and outcome. Variable outcomes are particularly frustrating to the pediatric intensivist who is faced with the reality that one patient with ARDS may survive, while another patient of similar age, having an identical trigger with seemingly similar comorbidities may die. These highly divergent outcomes may at times be explained by management strategies. However, recent progress in genomics suggests that part of the basis of these variable outcomes may lie in the genetic background of the child that predisposes him to more severe manifestation of ALI/ARDS.

The evolving field of genomics holds the promise of elucidating a genetic predisposition to ARDS and other diseases afflicting critically ill children.[187–189] Although no clear ARDS gene or marker has been established to date, there is good evidence that mutations, or polymorphisms, in surfactant protein genes can impart a phenotype characterized by the propensity to develop interstitial lung disease and/or ARDS.[190,191] In addition, polymorphisms of cytokine genes have been associated with increased mortality in sepsis, a primary cause of indirect ALI.[192,193]

Important tools for the application of genomics to the study of ARDS include the recent sequencing of the human genome, evolution of microarray technology, and expansion of powerful bioinformatics. With these tools it may become possible to further characterize the host response during ARDS at the genomic level. These studies are eagerly awaited because they hold the promise of increasing our understanding of ARDS with that hope that individual patients' responses can be more thoroughly characterized such that therapies can be more specifically tailored to the needs of the individual patient.

SUMMARY

ALI/ARDS continues to be a major cause of mortality in pediatric critical care medicine. It is clear that cytokines contribute to this pathophysiologic state via receptor-mediated signaling pathways that effect target cell responses. The application of molecular biology techniques into the field of critical care has both improved our understanding of this biological response and has identified a number of potential therapeutic targets. Although in vitro and animal model data have demonstrated the amelioration of the inflammatory response and lung injury by these strategies, the modalities that have been tested in humans thus far have proven ineffective. It is hoped that further understanding of the fundamental biology, improved identification of the patient's inflammatory state, and application of therapies directed at multiple sites of action may ultimately prove beneficial for patients suffering from ALI/ARDS.

FUTURE DIRECTIONS

Although use of adjuvant therapies is common in patients with ALI and ARDS, the only intervention that has proven to result in a significant mortality benefit in this population is a simple variation on a form of therapy required by all patients with this disease, regardless of etiology, namely, low V_T ventilation.[24] The low mortality now reported in pediatric ALI/ARDS trials may indicate the benefits of strictly protocolized, high-quality supportive care, but it also points out the challenges faced by clinical investigators when it comes to designing future trials with sufficient power to provide a reliable estimate of the effects of novel therapies in these diseases. Identifying additional opportunities to further improve outcomes in pediatric ALI/ARDS will likely depend on applying proven or promising therapies and care strategies at the earliest possible time in the disease process and clarifying which subgroups of ALI/ARDS patients stand to benefit from specific interventions.

REFERENCES

1. Ashbaugh D, Bigelow D, Petty T, et al. Acute respiratory distress in adults. Lancet 1967;2(7511):319–23.
2. Rubenfeld GD, Herridge MS. Epidemiology and outcomes of acute lung injury. Chest 2007;131(2):554–62.
3. Esteban A, Alia I, Gordo F, et al for the Spanish Lung Failure Collaborative Group. Prospective randomized trial comparing pressure-controlled ventilation and volume-controlled ventilation in ARDS. Chest 2000;117(6):1690–6.
4. Luhr OR, Antonsen K, Karlsson M, et al. Incidence and mortality after acute respiratory failure and acute respiratory distress syndrome in Sweden, Denmark, and Iceland: the ARF Study Group. Am J Respir Crit Care Med 1999;159(6):1849–61.
5. Zambon M., Vincent JL. Mortality rates for patients with acute lung injury/ARDS have decreased over time. Chest 2008;133(5):1120–7.
6. Matthay M. Conference summary: acute lung injury. Chest 1999;116(1 Suppl): 119–26.
7. Ware L, Matthay M. The acute respiratory distress syndrome. N Engl J Med 2000;342(18):1334–49.
8. Corbridge T, Wood L, Crawford G, et al. Adverse effects of large tidal volumes and low PEEP in canine acid aspiration. Am Rev Respir Dis 1990;142(2):311–5.
9. Dreyfuss D. Mechanical ventilation-induced pulmonary edema. Interaction with previous lung alterations. Am J Respir Crit Care Med 1995;151(5):1568–75.
10. Parker J, Townsley M, Rippe B, et al. Increased microvascular permeability in dog lungs due to high peak airway pressure. J Appl Physiol 1984;57(6):1809–16.
11. Slutsky A, Tremblay L. Multiple system organ failure: is mechanical ventilation a contributing factor? Am J Respir Crit Care Med 1998;157(6 Pt 1):1721–5.
12. Webb H, Tierney D. Experimental pulmonary edema due to intermittent positive pressure ventilation with high inflation pressures: protection by positive end-expiratory pressure. Am Rev Respir Dis 1974;110:556–61.
13. Demling R. The modern version of adult respiratory distress syndrome [review]. Ann Rev Med 1995;46:193–202.
14. Ingbar D. Acute respiratory distress syndrome: mechanisms of repair and remodeling following acute lung injury. Clin Chest Med 2000;21(3):589–616.
15. Lamy M, Fallat R, Koeniger E, et al. Pathologic features and mechanisms of hypoxemia in adult respiratory distress syndrome. Am Rev Respir Dis 1976;114: 267–71.
16. Tomashefski J Jr. Pulmonary pathology of the adult respiratory distress syndrome. Clin Chest Med 1990;11:593–619.
17. Baughman RP, Gunther KL, Rashkin MC, et al. Changes in the inflammatory response of the lung during acute respiratory distress syndrome: prognostic indicators. Am J Respir Crit Care Med 1996;154(1):76–81.
18. Meduri GU, Kohler G, Headley S, et al. Inflammatory cytokines in the BAL of patients with ARDS: persistent elevation over time predicts poor outcome. Chest 1995; 108(5):1303–14.

19. Dantzker D, Brook C, Dehart P, et al. Ventilation-perfusion distribution in the adult respiratory distress syndrome. Am Rev Respir Dis 1979;120:1039–45.
20. Ralph D, Robertson H, Weaver L, et al. Distribution of ventilation and perfusion during positive end-expiratory pressure in the adult respiratory distress syndrome. Am Rev Respir Dis 1985;131(1):54–60.
21. Montgomery A, Stager M, Carrico C, et al. Causes of mortality in patients with adult respiratory distress syndrome. Am Rev Respir Dis 1985;132(3):485–9.
22. Clark J, Milberg J, Steinberg K, et al. Type III procollagen peptide in adult respiratory distress syndrome: association of increased peptide levels in lavage fluid with increased risk of death. Ann Intern Med 1995;122(1):17–23.
23. Chesnutt AN, Matthay MA, Tibayan FA, et al. Early detection of type III procollagen peptide in acute lung injury: pathogenetic and prognostic significance. Am J Respir Crit Care Med 1997;156(3 Pt 1):840–5.
24. Brower RG, Matthay MA, Morris A, et al. Ventilation with lower tidal volumes as compared with traditional tidal volumes for acute lung injury and the acute respiratory distress syndrome. N Engl J Med 2000;342(18):1301–8.
25. Baughman R, Gunther K, Rashkin M, et al. Changes in the inflammatory response of the lung during acute respiratory distress syndrome: prognostic indicators. Am J Respir Crit Care Med 1996;154(1):76–81.
26. Luce J. Acute lung injury and the acute respiratory distress syndrome. Crit Care Med 1998;26(2):369–76.
27. Steinberg K, Hudson L. Acute lung injury and acute respiratory distress syndrome: the clinical syndrome. Clin Chest Med 2000;21(3):401–17.
28. Davidson T, Caldwell E, Curtis J, et al. Reduced quality of life in survivors of acute respiratory distress syndrome with critically ill control patients. JAMA 1999;281(4):354–60.
29. McHugh L, Milberg J, Whitcomb M, et al. Recovery of function in survivors of the acute respiratory distress syndrome. Am J Respir Crit Care Med 1994;150(1):90–4.
30. Schelling G, Stoll C, Hallar M. Health-related quality of life and posttraumatic disorder in survivors of acute respiratory distress syndrome. Crit Care Med 1998;26(4):651–9.
31. Weinert C, Gross C, Kangas J, et al. Health-related quality of life after acute lung injury. Am J Respir Crit Care Med 1997;156(4 Pt 1):1120–8.
32. Hopkins R, Weaver L, Pope D, et al. Neuropsychological sequelae and impaired health status in survivors of severe acute respiratory distress syndrome. Am J Respir Crit Care Med 1999;160(1):50–6.
33. Hopkins RO, Weaver LK, Collingridge D, et al. Two year cognitive, emotional and quality-of-life outcomes in acute respiratory distress syndrome. Am J Respir Crit Care Med 2005;171(4);340–7.
34. Dowdy DW, Dennison CR, Mendez-Tellez PA, et al. Quality of life after acute respiratory distress syndrome: a meta-analysis. Intensive Care Med 2006;32(8):1115–24.
35. Adhikari NKJ, Tansey C, McAndrews M, et al. Self-reported depressive symptoms and memory complaints in survivors five years after ARDS. Chest 2011;140(6):1484–93.
36. The ARDS Foundation. Gibbons M. Researchers need to study ARDS survivors after they leave the ICU. Available at: http://www.ardsusa.org. Accessed June 30, 2012.
37. Martin T. Lung cytokines and ARDS. Chest 1999;116(1 Suppl):2S–8S.
38. Papadakos P. Cytokines, genes, and ARDS. Chest 2002;121(5):1391–2.
39. Parsons P. Acute respiratory distress syndrome: mediators and mechanisms of acute lung injury. Clin Chest Med 2000;21(3):467–76.

40. Pugin J, Ricou B, Steinberg K, et al. Proinflammatory activity in bronchoalveolar lavage fluids from patients with ARDS, a prominent role for interleukin-1. Am J Respir Crit Care Med 1996;153(6 Pt 1):1850–6.

41. Pugin J, Verghese G, Widmer M-C, et al. The alveolar space is the site of intense inflammatory and profibrotic reactions in the early phase of acute respiratory distress syndrome. Crit Care Med 1999;27(2):304–12.

42. Strieter R, Kunkel S, Keane M, et al. Chemokines in lung injury. Chest 1999;116(1 Suppl):103S–5S.

43. Durbin CG, Wallace KK. Oxygen toxicity in the critically ill patient. Respir Care 1993;93(7):739–50.

44. Parker JC, Hernandez LA, Peevy KJ. Mechanisms of ventilator-induced lung injury. Crit Care Med 1993;21(1):131–43.

45. Dreyfuss D, Saumon G. Ventilator-induced lung injury: lessons from experimental studies. Am J Respir Crit Care Med 1998;157(1):294–323.

46. Murphy DB, Cregg N, Tremblay L, et al. Adverse ventilatory strategy causes pulmonary-to-systemic translocation of endotoxin. Am J Respir Crit Care Med 2000;162(1):27–33.

47. Tremblay L, Valenza F, Ribeiro SP, et al. Injurious ventilatory strategies increase cytokines and c-fos m-RNA expression in an isolated rat lung model. J Clin Invest 1997;99(5):944–52.

48. Tremblay LN, Slutsky AS. Ventilator-induced injury: from barotrauma to biotrauma. Proc Assoc Am Physicians 1998;110(6):482–8.

49. Vieillard-Baron A, Prin S, Augarde R, et al. Increasing respiratory rate to improve CO_2 clearance during mechanical ventilation is not a panacea in acute respiratory failure. Crit Care Med 2002;30(7):1407–12.

50. Arroliga AC, Thompson BT, Ancukiewicz M, et al, for the Acute Respiratory Distress Network. Use of sedatives, opioids, and neuromuscular blocking agents in patients with acute lung injury and acute respiratory distress syndrome. Crit Care Med 2008;36(4):1083–8.

51. Papazian L, Forel JM, Gacouin A, et al. Neuromuscular blockers in early acute respiratory distress syndrome. N Engl J Med 2010;363(16):1107–16.

52. Slutsky AS. Neuromuscular blocking agents in ARDS. N Engl J Med 2010;363(12): 1176–80.

53. Esan A, Hess DR, Raoof S, et al. Severe hypoxemic respiratory failure: part 1—ventilatory strategies. Chest 2010;137(5):1203–16.

54. Brower RG, Lanken PN, MacIntryre N, et al. Higher versus lower positive end-expiratory pressures in patients with the acute respiratory distress syndrome. N Eng J Med 2004;351(4):327–36.

55. Ramnath VR, Hess DR, Thompson BT. Conventional mechanical ventilation in acute lung injury and acute respiratory distress syndrome. Clin Chest Med 2006;27(4): 601–13.

56. Lachmann B. Open the lung and keep the lung open. Intensive Care Med 1992; 18(6):319–21.

57. Lachmann B. Open lung in ARDS. Minerva Anesthesiol 2002;68(9):637–42.

58. Amato MBP, Barbas CSV, Medeiros DM, et al. Effect of a protective-ventilation strategy on mortality in the acute respiratory distress syndrome. N Engl J Med 1998;338(6):347–54.

59. Villar J, Kacmarek RM, Perez-Mendez L, et al for the ARIES Network. A high positive end-expiratory pressure, low tidal volume ventilation strategy improves outcome in persistent acute respiratory distress syndrome: a randomized, controlled trial. Crit Care Med 2006;34(5):1311–8.

60. Albaiceta GM, Luyando LH, Parra D, et al. Inspiratory vs expiratory pressure-volume curves to set end-expiratory pressure in acute lung injury. Intensive Care Med 2005;31(10):1370–8.

61. Caramez MP, Kacmarek RM, Helmy M, et al. A comparison of methods to identify open-lung PEEP. Intensive Care Med 2009;35(4):740–7.

62. Ranieri VM, Zhang H, Mascia L, et al. Pressure-time curve predicts minimally injurious ventilatory strategy in an isolated rat lung model. Anesthesiol 2000;93(5):1320–8.

63. Grasso S, Terragni P, Mascia L, et al. Airway pressure-time curve profile (stress-index) detects tidal recruitment/hyperinflation in experimental acute lung injury. Crit Care Med 2004;32(4):1018–27.

64. Formenti P, Graf J, Santos A, et al. Non-pulmonary factors strongly influence the stress index. Intensive Care Med 2011;37(4):594–600.

65. Talmor D, Sarge T, Malhotra A, et al. Mechanical ventilation guided by esophageal pressure in acute lung injury. N Engl J Med 2008;359(20):2095–104.

66. Talmor DS, Fessler HE. Are esophageal pressure measurements important in clinical decision-making in mechanically ventilated patients? Respir Care 2010;55(2):162–72.

67. Loring SH, O'Donnell CR, Behazin N, et al. Esophageal pressures in acute lung injury: do they represent artifact or useful information about transpulmonary pressure, chest wall mechanics, and lung stress? J Appl Physiol 2010;108(3):515–22.

68. Richard JCM, Marini JJ. Transpulmonoary pressure as a surrogate of plateau pressure for lung protective strategy: not perfect but more physiologic. Intensive Care Med 2012;38(3):339–41.

69. Meade MO, Cook DJ, Guyatt GH, et al. Ventilation strategy using low tidal volumes, recruitment maneuvers, and high positive end-expiratory pressure for acute lung injury and acute respiratory distress syndrome: a randomized clinical trial. JAMA 2008;299(6):637–45.

70. Mercat A, Richard JCM, Vielle B, et al. Positive end-expiratory pressure setting in adults with acute lung injury and acute respiratory distress syndrome: a randomized controlled trial. JAMA 2008;299(6):646–55.

71. Briel M, Meade M, Mercat A, et al. Higher vs lower positive end-expiratory pressure in patients with acute lung injury and acute respiratory distress syndrome. JAMA 2010;303(9):865–73.

72. Fan E, Wilcox ME, Brower RG, et al. Recruitment maneuvers for acute lung injury: a systematic review. Am J Respir Crit Care Med 2008;178(11):1156–63.

73. Kacmarek RM, Villar J. Lung recruitment maneuvers during acute respiratory distress syndrome: is it useful? Minerva Anestesiol 2011;77(1):85–9.

74. Iannuzzi M, De Sio A, De Robertis E, et al. Different patterns of lung recruitment maneuvers in primary acute respiratory distress syndrome: effects on oxygenation and central hemodynamics. Minerva Anestesiol 2010;76(9):692–8.

75. Arnal JM, Paquet J, Wysocki M, et al. Optimal duration of a sustained inflation recruitment maneuver in ARDS patients. Intensive Care Med 2011;37(10):1588–94.

76. Rocco PR, Pelosi P, de Abreu P. Pros and cons of recruitment maneuvers in acute lung injury and acute respiratory distress syndrome. Expert Rev Respir Med 2010;4(4):479–89.

77. Downs JB, Stock MC. Airway pressure release ventilation: a new concept in ventilatory support. Crit Care Med 1987;15(5):459–61.

78. Stock MC, Downs JB, Frolicher DA. Airway pressure release ventilation. Crit Care Med 1987;15(5):462–6.

79. Habashi NM. Other approaches to open-lung ventilation: airway pressure release ventilation. Crit Care Med 2005;33(3 Suppl):S228–S240.

80. Putensen C, Zech S, Wrigge H, et al. Long-term effects of spontaneous breathing during ventilatory support in patients with acute lung injury. Am J Respir Crit Care Med 2001;164(1):43–9.
81. Hedenstierna G, Lichtwarck-Aschoff M. Interfacing spontaneous breathing and mechnical ventilation. Minerva Anesthesiol 2006;72(4):183–98.
82. Rasanen J, Cane RD, Downs JB, et al. Airway pressure release ventilation during acute lung injury: a prospective multicenter trial. Crit Care Med 1991;19(10):1234–41.
83. Davis K, Johnson DJ, Branson RD, et al. Airway pressure release ventilation. Arch Surg 1993;128(12):1348–52.
84. Dart BW, Maxwell RA, Richart CM, et al. Preliminary experience with airway pressure release ventilation in a trauma/surgical intensive care unit. J Trauma 2005;59(1):71–6.
85. Liu L, Tanigawa K, Ota K, et al. Practical use of airway pressure release ventilation for severe ARDS—a preliminary report in comparison with a conventional ventilatory support. Hiroshima J Med Sci 2009;58(4):83–8.
86. Varpula T, Valta P, Niemi R, et al. Airway pressure release ventilation as a primary ventilatory mode in acute respiratory distress syndrome. Acta Anaesthesiol Scand 2004;48(6):722–31.
87. Varpula T, Valta P, Markkola A, et al. The effects of ventilatory mode on lung aeration assessed with computer tomography: a randomized controlled study. J Intensive Care Med 2009;24(2):122–30.
88. Maxwell RA, Green JM, Waldrop J, et al. A randomized prospective trial of airway pressure release ventilation and low tidal volume ventilation in adult trauma patients with acute respiratory failure. J Trauma 2010;69:501–11.
89. Imai I, Slutsky AS. High-frequency oscillatory ventilation and ventilator-induced lung injury. Crit Care Med 2005;33(3 Suppl):S129–S34.
90. Hager DN, Fessler HE, Kaczka DW, et al. Tidal volume delivery during high-frequency oscillatory ventilation in adults with acute respiratory distress syndrome. Crit Care Med 2007;35(6):1522–9.
91. Rotta AT, Gunnarsson B, Fuhrman BP, et al. Comparison of lung protective ventilation strategies in a rabbit model of acute lung injury. Crit Care Med 2001;29(11):2176–84.
92. Hamilton PP, Onayemi A, Smyth JA, et al. Comparison of conventional and high frequency ventilation: oxygenation and lung pathology. J Appl Physiol 1983;55(1):131–8.
93. Muellenbach RM, Kredel M, Said HM, et al. High-frequency oscillatory ventilation reduces lung inflammation: a large-animal 24-h model of respiratory distress. Intensive Care Med 2007;33(8):1423–33.
94. Imai Y, Nakagawa S, Ito Y, et al. Comparison of lung protection strategies using conventional and high-frequency oscillatory ventilation. J Appl Physiol 2001;91(4):1836–44.
95. Fort P, Farmer C, Westerman J, et al. High-frequency oscillatory ventilation for adult respiratory distress syndrome-a pilot study. Crit Care Med 1997;25(6):937–47.
96. Mehta S, Lapinsky SE, Hallett DC, et al. Prospective trial of high-frequency oscillation in adults with acute respiratory distress syndrome. Crit Care Med 2001;29(7):1360–9.
97. Anderson FA, Guttormsen AB, Flaatten HK. High frequency oscillatory ventilation in adult patients with acute respiratory distress syndrome—a retrospective study. Acta Anaesthesiol Scand 2002;46(9):1082–8.
98. David M, Weiler N, Heinrichs W, et al. High-frequency oscillatory ventilation in adult acute respiratory distress syndrome. Intensive Care Med 2003;29(10):1656–65.

99. Cartotto R, Ellis S, Gomez M, et al. High frequency oscillatory ventilation in burn patients with the acute respiratory distress syndrome. Burns 2004;30(5):453–63.
100. Ferguson ND, Chiche JD, Kacmarek RM, et al. Combining high-frequency oscillatory ventilation and recruitment maneuvers in adults with early respiratory distress syndrome: the treatment with oscillation and an open lung strategy (TOOLS) trial pilot study. Crit Care Med 2005;33(3):479–86.
101. Pachl J, Roubik K, Waldauf P, et al. Normocapnic high-frequency oscillatory ventilation affects differently extrapulmonary and pulmonary forms of acute respiratory distress syndrome in adults. Physiol Res 2006;55(1):15–24.
102. Finkielman JD, Gajic O, Farmer JC, et al. The initial Mayo Clinic experience using high-frequency oscillatory ventilation for adult patients: a retrospective study. BMC Emerg Med 2006;6(2):1–8.
103. Kao KC, Tsai YH, Wu YK, et al. High frequency oscillatory ventilation for surgical patients with acute respiratory distress syndrome. J Trauma 2006;61(4):837–43.
104. Derdak S, Mehta S, Stewart TE, et al. High-frequency oscillatory ventilation for acute respiratory distress syndrome in adults: a randomized, controlled trial. Am J Respir Crit Care Med 2002;166(6):801–8.
105. Bollen CW, van Well GTJ, Sherry T, et al. High frequency oscillatory ventilation compared with conventional mechanical ventilation in adult respiratory distress syndrome: a randomized controlled trial. Crit Care 2005;9:R430–9.
106. Papazian L, Gainnier M, Marin V, et al. Comparison of prone positioning and high-frequency oscillatory ventilation in patients with acute respiratory distress syndrome. Crit Care Med 2005;33(10):2162–71.
107. Demory D, Michelet P, Arnal JM, et al. High frequency oscillatory ventilation following prone positioning prevents a further impairment in oxygenation. Crit Care Med 2007;35(1):106–11.
108. Fessler HE, Derdak S, Ferguson ND, et al. A protocol for high-frequency oscillatory ventilation in adults: results from a roundtable discussion. Crit Care Med 2007;35(7):1649–54.
109. Fessler HE, Hager DN, Brower RG. Feasibility of very high-frequency ventilation in adults with acute respiratory distress syndrome. Crit Care Med 2008;36(4):1043–8.
110. Griffiths MJ, Evans TW. Inhaled nitric oxide therapy in adults. N Engl J Med 2005;353(25):2683–95.
111. Payen DM. Inhaled nitric oxide and acute lung injury. Clin Chest Med 2000;21(3):519–29, ix.
112. Puybasset L, Rouby JJ. Pulmonary uptake and modes of administration of inhaled nitric oxide in mechanically-ventilated patients. Crit Care 1998;2:9–17.
113. Rossaint R, Falke KJ, Lopez F, et al. Inhaled nitric oxide for the adult respiratory distress syndrome. N Engl J Med 1993;328(6):399–405.
114. Adnot S, Raffestin B, Eddahibi S. NO in the lung. Respir Physiol 1995;101(2):109–20.
115. Pison U, Lopez FA, Heidelmeyer CF, et al. Inhaled nitric oxide reverses hypoxic pulmonary vasoconstriction without impairing gas exchange. J Appl Physiol 1993;74:1287–92.
116. Creagh-Brown BC, Griffiths MJ, Evans TW. Bench-to-bedside review: inhaled nitric oxide therapy in adults. Crit Care 2009;13(3):221.
117. Dellinger RP, Zimmerman JL, Taylor RW, et al for Inhaled Nitric Oxide in ARDS Study Group. Effects of inhaled nitric oxide in patients with acute respiratory distress syndrome: results of a randomized phase II trial. Crit Care Med 1998;26(1):15–23.

118. Troncy E, Collet JP, Shapiro S, et al. Inhaled nitric oxide in acute respiratory distress syndrome: a pilot randomized controlled study. Am J Respir Crit Care Med 1998; 157(5 Pt 1):1483–8.

119. Michael JR, Barton RG, Saffle JR, et al. Inhaled nitric oxide versus conventional therapy: effect on oxygenation in ARDS. Am J Respir Crit Care Med 1998;157(5 Pt 1):1372–80.

120. Taylor RW, Zimmerman JL, Dellinger RP, et al. Low-dose inhaled nitric oxide in patients with acute lung injury: a randomized controlled trial. JAMA 2004;291(13): 1603–9.

121. Lundin S, Mang H, Smithies M, et al for The European Study Group of Inhaled Nitric Oxide. Inhalation of nitric oxide in acute lung injury: results of a European multicentre study. Intensive Care Med 1999;25(9):911–9.

122. Adhikari NK, Burns KE, Friedrich JO, et al. Effect of nitric oxide on oxygenation and mortality in acute lung injury: systematic review and meta-analysis. BMJ 2007; 334(7597):779.

123. Abman SH, Griebel JL, Parker DK, et al. Acute effects of inhaled nitric oxide in children with severe hypoxemic respiratory failure. J Pediatr 1994;124(6):881–8.

124. Dobyns EL, Cornfield DN, Anas NG, et al. Multicenter randomized controlled trial of the effects of inhaled nitric oxide therapy on gas exchange in children with acute hypoxemic respiratory failure. J Pediatr 1999;134(4):406–12.

125. Dobyns EL, Anas NG, Fortenberry JD, et al. Interactive effects of high-frequency oscillatory ventilation and inhaled nitric oxide in acute hypoxemic respiratory failure in pediatrics. Crit Care Med 2002;30(11):2425–9.

126. Warren JB, Higenbottam T. Caution with use of inhaled nitric oxide. Lancet 1996; 348(9028):629–30.

127. Quinn AC, Petros AJ, Vallance P. Nitric oxide: an endogenous gas. Br J Anaesth 1995;74(4):443–51.

128. Zabrocki LA, Brogan TV, Statler KD, et al. Extracorporeal membrane oxygenation for pediatric respiratory failure: survival and predictors of mortality. Crit Care Med 2011;39(2):364–70.

129. Moler FW, Palmisano JM, Green TP, et al. Predictors of outcome of severe respiratory syncytial virus-associated respiratory failure treated with extracorporeal membrane oxygenation. J Pediatr 1993;123(1):46–52.

130. Green TP, Moler FW, Goodman DM for Extracorporeal Life Support Organization. Probability of survival after prolonged extracorporeal membrane oxygenation in pediatric patients with acute respiratory failure. Crit Care Med 1995;23(6):1132–9.

131. Pranikoff T, Hirschl RB, Steimle CN, et al. Mortality is directly related to the duration of mechanical ventilation before the initiation of extracorporeal life support for severe respiratory failure. Crit Care Med 1997;25(1):28–32.

132. Arnold JH, Hanson JH, Toro-Figuero LO, et al. Prospective, randomized comparison of high-frequency oscillatory ventilation and conventional mechanical ventilation in pediatric respiratory failure. Crit Care Med 1994;22(10):1530–9.

133. Trachsel D, McCrindle BW, Nakagawa S, et al. Oxygenation index predicts outcome in children with acute hypoxemic respiratory failure. Am J Respir Crit Care Med 2005;172(2):206–11.

134. Hemmila MR, Rowe SA, Boules TN, et al. Extracorporeal life support for severe acute respiratory distress syndrome in adults. Ann Surg 2004;240(4):595–605 [discussion: 605–7].

135. Rollins MD, Hubbard A, Zabrocki L, et al. Extracorporeal membrane oxygenation cannulation trends for pediatric respiratory failure and central nervous system injury. J Pediatr Surg 2012;47:68–75.

136. Zahraa JN, Moler FW, Annich GM, et al. Venovenous versus venoarterial extracorporeal life support for pediatric respiratory failure: are there differences in survival and acute complications? Crit Care Med 2000;28(2):521–5.

137. Peek GJ, Mugford M, Tiruvoipati R, et al. Efficacy and economic assessment of conventional ventilatory support versus extracorporeal membrane oxygenation for severe adult respiratory failure (CESAR): a multicentre randomised controlled trial. Lancet 2009;374(9698):1351–63.

138. Ware LB, Matthay MA. Alveolar fluid clearance is impaired in the majority of patients with acute lung injury and the acute respiratory distress syndrome. Am J Respir Crit Care Med 2001;163(6):1376–83.

139. Pittet JF, Wiener-Kronish JP, McElroy MC, et al. Stimulation of lung epithelial liquid clearance by endogenous release of catecholamines in septic shock in anesthetized rats. J Clin Invest 1994;94(2):663–71.

140. Perkins GD, McAuley DF, Thickett DR, et al. The beta-agonist lung injury trial (BALTI): a randomized placebo-controlled clinical trial. Am J Respir Crit Care Med 2006; 173(3):281–7.

141. Perkins GD, McAuley DF. Pro: beta-agonists in acute lung injury—the end of the story? Am J Respir Crit Care Med 2011;184(5):503–4.

142. Papazian L. Con: beta$_2$–adrenergic agonists in ALI/ARDS—not recommended or potentially harmful? Am J Respir Crit Care Med 2011;184(5):504–6.

143. Thompson BT. Beta-agonists for ARDS: the dark side of adrenergic stimulation? Lancet 2012;379:196–8.

144. Matthay MA, Brower RG, Carson S, et al. Randomized, placebo-controlled clinical trial of an aerosolized beta-agonist for treatment of acute lung injury. Am J Respir Crit Care Med 2011;184(5):561–8.

145. Au DH, Curtis JR, Every NR, et al. Association between inhaled beta-agonists and the risk of unstable angina and myocardial infarction. Chest 2002;121(3):846–51.

146. Modelska K, Matthay MA, Brown LA, et al. Inhibition of beta-adrenergic-dependent alveolar epithelial clearance by oxidant mechanisms after hemorrhagic shock. Am J Physiol 1999;276(5 Pt 1):L844–57.

147. Frank JA, Pittet JF, Lee H, et al. High tidal volume ventilation induces NOS2 and impairs cAMP-dependent air space fluid clearance. Am J Physiol Lung Cell Mol Physiol 2003;284(5):L791–8.

148. Sartori C, Allemann Y, Duplain H, et al. Salmeterol for the prevention of high-altitude pulmonary edema. N Engl J Med 2002;346(21):1631–6.

149. Licker M, Tschopp JM, Robert J, et al. Aerosolized salbutamol accelerates the resolution of pulmonary edema after lung resection. Chest 2008;133(4):845–52.

150. Perkins GD, Park D, Alderson D, et al. The Beta Agonist Lung Injury Trial (BALTI)—prevention trial protocol. Trials 2011;12:79.

151. Ware LB, Koyama T, Billheimer D, et al. Advancing donor management research: design and implementation of a large, randomized, placebo-controlled trial. Ann Intensive Care 2011;1:20.

152. Stern M, Ulrich K, Robinson C, et al. Pretreatment with cationic lipid-mediated transfer of the Na^+K^+-ATPase pump in a mouse model in vivo augments resolution of high permeability pulmonary oedema. Gene Ther 2000;7(11):960–6.

153. Luster AD, Alon R, von Andrian UH. Immune cell migration in inflammation: present and future therapeutic targets. Nat Immunol 2005;6:1182–90.

154. Lawrence MB, Springer TA. Leukocytes roll on a selectin at physiologic flow rates: distinction from and prerequisite for adhesion through integrins. Cell 1991;65:859–73.

155. Butcher EC. Leukocyte-endothelial cell recognition: three (or more) steps to specificity and diversity. Cell 1991;67:1033–6.
156. Orlova VV, Chavakis T. Regulation of vascular endothelial permeability by junctional adhesion molecules (JAM). Thromb Haemost 2007;98:327–32.
157. Ley K, Laudanna C, Cybulsky MI, et al. Getting to the site of inflammation: the leuhocyte adhesion cascade update. Nat Rev Immunol 2007;7:678–89.
158. Rao RM, Yang L, Garcia-Cardena G, et al. Endothelial-dependent mechanisms of leukocyte recruitment to the vascular wall. Circ Res 2007;101:234–7.
159. Schenekl AR, Mamdouh Z, Muller WA. Locomotion of monocytes on endothelium is a critical step suring extravasation. Nat Immunol 2004;5:393–400.
160. Imhof BA, Aurrand-Lions M. Adhesion mechanisms regulating the migration of monocytes. Nat Rev Immunol 2004;4:432–44.
161. Kinashi T. Intracellular signalling controlling integrin activation in lymphocytes. Nat Rev Immunol 2005;5:546–59.
162. Vestweber D. Adhesion and signalling molecules controlling the transmigration of leukocytes through endothelium. Immunol Rev 2007;218:178–96.
163. Springer TA. Traffic signals for lymphocyte recirculation and leukocyte emigration: the multistep paradigm. Cell 1994;76:301–14.
164. Kumasaka T, Quinlan WM, Doyle NA, et al. Role of the intercellular adhesion molecule-1(ICAM-1) in endotoxin-induced pneumonia evaluated using ICAM-1 antisense oligonucleotides, anti-ICAM-1 monoclonal antibodies, and ICAM-1 mutant mice. J Clin Invest 1996;97:2362–9.
165. Doerschuk CM, Quinlan WM, Doyle NA, et al. The role of P-selectin and ICAM-1 in acute lung injury as determined using blocking antibodies and mutant mice. J Immunol 1996;157(10):4609–14.
166. Ridings PC, Windsor AC, Jutila MA, et al. A dual-binding antibody to E- and L-selectin attenuates sepsis-induced lung injury. Am J Respir Crit Care Med 1995;152(1):247–53.
167. Mulligan MS, Miyasaka M, Tamatani T, et al. Requirements for L-selectin in neutrophil-mediated lung injury in rats. J Immunol 1994;152(2):832–40.
168. Mulligan MS, Polley MJ, Bayer RJ, et al. Neutrophil-dependent acute lung injury: requirement for P-selectin (GMP-140). J Clin Invest 1992;90(4):1600–7.
169. Etzioni A, Alon R. Leukocyte adhesion deficiency III: a group of integrin activation defects in hematopoietic lineage cells. Curr Opin Allergy Clin Immunol 2004;4(6):485–90.
170. Kinashi T, Aker M, Sokolovsky-Eisenberg M, et al. LAD-III, a leukocyte adhesion deficiency syndrome associated with defective Rap1 activation and impaired stabilization of integrin bonds. Blood 2004;103(3):1033–6.
171. Bogdan C, Vodovotz Y, Nathan C. Macrophage deactivation by interleukin 10. J Exp Med 1991;174(6):1549–55.
172. Bogdan C, Paik J, Vodovotz Y, et al. Contrasting mechanisms for suppression of macrophage cytokine release by transforming growth factor-beta and interleukin-10. J Biol Chem 1992;267(32):23301–8.
173. DeVries A, Semchuk WM, Betcher JG. Ketoconazole in the prevention of acute respiratory distress syndrome. Pharmacotherapy 1998;18(3):581–7.
174. Williams JG, Maier RV. Ketoconazole inhibits alveolar macrophage production of inflammatory mediators involved in acute lung injury (adult respiratory distress syndrome). Surgery 1992;112(2):270–7.
175. The ARDS Clinical Trials Network, National Heart Lung, and Blood Institute, National Institutes of Health. Randomized, placebo-controlled trial of lisofylline for early treatment of acute lung injury and acute respiratory distress syndrome. Crit Care Med 2002;30:1–6.
176. Bone RC. Why sepsis trials fail. JAMA 1996;276(7):565–6.

177. Fisher CJ Jr, Agosti JM, Opal SM, et al for the Soluble TNF Receptor Sepsis Study Group. Treatment of septic shock with the tumor necrosis factor receptor:Fc fusion protein. N Engl J Med 1996;334:1697–702.
178. Lemeshow S, Teres D, Moseley S. Statistical issues in clinical sepsis trials. Baltimore (MD): Williams & Wilkins; 1996.
179. Yanik GA, Ho VT, Levine JE, et al. The impact of soluble tumor necrosis factor receptor etanercept on the treatment of idiopathic pneumonia syndrome after allogeneic hematopoietic stem cell transplantation. Blood 2008;112(8):3073–81.
180. Panoskaltsis-Mortari A, Griese M, Madtes DK, et al. An official American Thoracic Society research statement: noninfectious lung injury after hematopoietic stem cell transplantation: idiopathic pneumonia syndrome. Am J Respir Crit Care Med 2011; 183(9):1262–79.
181. Matsumoto T, Yokoi K, Mukaida N, et al. Pivotal role of interleukin-8 in the acute respiratory distress syndrome and cerebral reperfusion injury. J Leukoc Biol 1997; 62(5):581–7.
182. Folkesson HG, Matthay MA, Hebert CA, et al. Acid aspiration-induced lung injury in rabbits is mediated by interleukin-8-dependent mechanisms. J Clin Invest 1995; 96(1):107–16.
183. Mulligan MS, Jones ML, Bolanowski MA, et al. Inhibition of lung inflammatory reactions in rats by an anti-human IL-8 antibody. J Immunol 1993;150(12):5585–95.
184. Kurdowska A, Noble JM, Steinberg KP, et al. Anti-interleukin 8 autoantibody: interleukin 8 complexes in the acute respiratory distress syndrome. Relationship between the complexes and clinical disease activity. Am J Respir Crit Care Med 2001;163(2):463–8.
185. Krupa A, Kato H, Matthay MA, et al. Proinflammatory activity of anti-IL-8 autoantibody:IL-8 complexes in alveolar edema fluid from patients with acute lung injury. Am J Physiol Lung Cell Mol Physiol 2004;286(6):L1105–13.
186. Ponath PD. Chemokine receptor antagonists: novel therapeutics for inflammation and AIDS. Expert Opin Invest Drugs 1998;7:1–18.
187. Mehta NM, Arnold JH. Genetic polymorphisms in acute respiratory distress syndrome: new approach to an old problem. Crit Care Med 2005;33(10):2443–5.
188. Floros J, Pavlovic J. Genetics of acute respiratory distress syndrome: challenges, approaches, surfactant proteins as candidate genes. Semin Respir Crit Care Med 2003;24(2):161–8.
189. Shanley TP, Wong HR. Molecular genetics in the pediatric intensive care unit. Crit Care Clin 2003;19(3):577–94.
190. Lin Z, Pearson C, Chinchilli V, et al. Polymorphisms of human SP-A, SP-B, and SP-D genes: association of SP-B Thr131Ile with ARDS. Clin Genet 2000;58(6):181–91.
191. Nogee LM, Dunbar AE 3rd, Wert SE, et al. A mutation in the surfactant protein C gene associated with familial interstitial lung disease. N Engl J Med 2001;344(8): 573–9.
192. Stuber F, Petersen M, Bokelmann F, et al. A genomic polymorphism within the tumor necrosis factor locus influences plasma tumor necrosis factor-alpha concentrations and outcome of patients with severe sepsis. Crit Care Med 1996;24(2):381–4.
193. Mira JP, Cariou A, Grall F, et al. Association of TNF2, a TNF-alpha promoter polymorphism, with septic shock susceptibility and mortality: a multicenter study. JAMA 1999;282(6):561–8.

Pulmonary Complications of Transfused Blood Components

Alexander B. Benson, MD

KEYWORDS

- Blood component transfusion • Blood transfusion • Red blood cell transfusion
- Acute lung injury • Pulmonary edema • Critical care

KEY POINTS

- There are potentially fatal complications of blood transfusion involving both transfusion-specific and patient-specific factors.
- Transfused blood components should be administered only after careful consideration of the patient's unique risk of a transfusion complication versus the physiologic benefit of the planned transfused blood component.
- Blood components should be treated like pharmaceuticals, with continued refinement of the product in response to common and deadly side effects and large multicenter trials performed to demonstrate efficacy. In the meantime, with regard to transfusion, less is often more.

INTRODUCTION

T ransfusion is common in critically ill patients, with up to 44% of patients admitted to an intensive care unit (ICU) in the United States receiving a transfusion.[1] Red blood cell transfusions are given most commonly due to anemia in both bleeding and nonbleeding patients, whereas platelets or plasma should be utilized primarily in bleeding patients, or before surgeries or procedures in which microvascular bleeding complications are probable because of quantitative or qualitative platelet abnormalities or coagulation imbalances.[1]

Three transfusion complications are responsibility for the majority of morbidity and mortality associated with transfused blood components in hospitalized patients. The respiratory complications associated with these pathophysiologic processes are discussed, including definitions, diagnosis, mechanism, incidence, risk factors, clinical management, and strategies for prevention. In addition, this article explores how different patient populations and different blood components differentially affect

This work was supported by grant no. K24 HLO89223 from the National Institutes of Health. The author has nothing to disclose.
Division of Pulmonary Sciences and Critical Care Medicine, University of Colorado Denver, 12700 East 19th Avenue, Aurora, CO 80045, USA
E-mail address: alexander.benson@ucdenver.edu

the risk of these deadly transfusion complications. Lastly, the article discusses how health care providers can risk-stratify individual patients or patient populations to determine whether a given transfusion is more likely to benefit or harm the patient based on the transfusion indication, risk, and expected result.

The "terrible T's" refer to transfusion-related acute lung injury (TRALI), transfusion-associated circulatory overload (TACO), and transfusion-related immunomodulation (TRIM). These transfusion complications primarily damage the lung, leading to respiratory failure. In addition, these potential complications are not commonly addressed during consent for blood components, but lead to significant patient morbidity and mortality, especially in critically ill and postoperative patient populations. TRALI is the most extensively studied of these three conditions; therefore a description of this condition is more extensive than that of TACO or TRIM.

TRALI

The consensus conference definition of TRALI is new acute lung injury occurring during or within 6 hours after a transfusion, with a clear temporal relationship to the transfusion.[2] TRALI has become the leading cause of transfusion-related mortality in most of the industrialized world.[3-7] In 1983, Popovsky and colleagues from the Mayo Clinic described five cases of noncardiogenic pulmonary edema after transfusion of packed red blood cells (PRBCs) or whole blood and coined the term TRALI to describe this syndrome.[8]

Diagnosis of TRALI

In 2004, the National Heart, Lung, and Blood Institute convened a working group to identify a common clinical definition to promote research in TRALI. The diagnosis must satisfy the criteria for acute lung injury (ALI), including (1) acute onset, (2) hypoxemic lung disease with (3) bilateral infiltrates on frontal chest radiograph, and (4) no evidence of left atrial hypertension (**Table 1**).[9] If an arterial blood gas is not available, an oxygen saturation (SPO_2) of 90% or less meets the acute hypoxemia criterion when a patient is breathing room air at sea level.[2]

In addition to meeting the standard criteria for ALI, TRALI requires further criteria (see **Table 1**). A patient must develop ALI during or within 6 hours of transfusion and no ALI may be present before transfusion. If alternative ALI risk factors exist (ie, sepsis, trauma, aspiration), TRALI can still be diagnosed if the clinical course of the patient suggests that ALI resulted mechanistically from the transfusion alone or a synergistic relationship between the transfusion and the underlying risk factor. If the temporal relationship between the transfusion and ALI (within 6 hours) is considered coincidental to the development of ALI from an alternate risk factor, a diagnosis of TRALI should not be used.[2] Laboratory findings are not included as diagnostic criteria for TRALI; however, transient acute leukopenia, leukocyte antigen–antibody match between donor and recipient (HLA class I or II, anti-granulocyte or anti-monocyte), or increased neutrophil priming activity in the plasma of blood products have been described and support the diagnosis of TRALI.[2]

Differentiating TRALI from Other Pulmonary-Related Transfusion Complications

The differential diagnosis for patients who develop respiratory distress during or within a few hours after transfusion include TRALI, TACO, an anaphylactic transfusion reaction, and transfusion of contaminated (bacteria) blood products. Differentiating these four syndromes is difficult due to similarities in their clinical presentation. Pulmonary complications of TRIM are delayed, so this transfusion complication is not considered in the context of an acute onset.

Table 1
Diagnostic criteria for transfusion-related acute lung injury (TRALI)

Consensus definition of ALI	
Timing:	Acute in onset
Hypoxemia:	$Pao_2/Fio_2 \leq 300$ OR $SPo_2 <90\%$ at sea level on room air
Chest radiograph:	Bilateral infiltrates seen on frontal chest radiograph
Edema not purely hydrostatic	No clinical evidence of left atrial hypertension
Consensus definition of TRALI (ALI diagnosis + three criteria below)	
1. Onset of signs or symptoms ≤ 6 h after transfusion	
2. ALI not present before transfusion	
3. Alternative ALI risk factors may be present; clinical course should determine whether the ALI is mechanistically related to the transfusion.	
Transient leukopenia, fever, hypotension may be present (not required).	

Differentiating TRALI (permeability pulmonary edema) from TACO (hydrostatic pulmonary edema) is difficult in the setting of underlying heart failure, renal failure, massive transfusion, or resuscitation.[10] In both syndromes the acute onset of pulmonary edema results in severe dyspnea, tachypnea, and worsening or new hypoxemia. Transient neutropenia may support the diagnosis of TRALI due to neutrophil sequestration in the lung, but if not present it does not rule out TRALI.[11] TRALI is more commonly associated with relative hypotension while TACO results in relative hypertension from pre-transfusion to post-transfusion. Clinical factors differentiating TACO from TRALI include distended neck veins, S3 on cardiac examination, and peripheral edema consistent with volume overload. A chest radiograph with septal lines, cephalisation, and an enlarged vascular pedicle (>65 mm) is more consistent with TACO. The most important clinical determinant of TACO is the rapid resolution time of the patient's pulmonary edema after successfully reducing pulmonary capillary pressures through diuresis. Antibody testing of the implicated blood components lacks sensitivity for TRALI because non-antibody–mediated mechanisms are common. However, testing is still recommended and may be helpful if antibody levels are detected.

Unlike TRALI and TACO, anaphylactic transfusion reactions usually present with bronchospasm rather than pulmonary edema. As a result, wheezing rather than crackles are heard during pulmonary auscultation and a clear chest radiograph rather than new infiltrates will accompany the respiratory distress. Similar to TRALI, fever and vasodilatory shock is common with anaphylaxis, but erythema and edema with associated urticaria over the head, neck, and trunk is more consistent with anaphylaxis.[12] Lastly, the transfusion of contaminated PRBCs or platelet concentrates may result in transfusion-related bacterial sepsis that manifests as septic shock and acute lung injury. Transfusion-related bacterial sepsis must be considered if septic shock is the overriding clinical presentation, and culturing the component bags is essential for diagnosis.[12]

Mechanism of TRALI

Multiple animal studies as well as epidemiologic and translational observations in humans with TRALI support a two-event mechanism. First, the pulmonary vascular endothelium is activated resulting in neutrophil "priming" and adhesion within the pulmonary microvasculature. Many different clinical states can trigger this "first event" (ie, sepsis, surgery, trauma, systemic inflammatory state). These primed, sequestered neutrophils are hyperactive and easily activated by a "second event." Identified triggers in blood components known to induce a "second event" and subsequent TRALI in humans and animals include donor antibodies to recipient leukocyte antigens, bioactive lipids, soluble CD40-ligand, microparticles, and others.[13,14] Animals develop TRALI after transfusion of blood components with high concentrations of known TRALI mediators (second event) only when administered lipopolysaccharide (first event) before transfusion.[15,16] In rare situations, a "first event" is not required because certain antibody–antigen interactions (most commonly HNA-3a, an anti-neutrophil antibody) from blood components alone have enough activation energy to trigger the whole chain of events.[17]

Multiple disease processes are capable of activating the pulmonary vascular endothelium and inducing adherence of neutrophils.[17] The higher incidence of TRALI in ICU patients (8%), as compared to a mixed population of hospitalized patients (0.16%) at the same institution, is likely a result of the "primed" state induced by critical illness.[18,19]

The Incidence of TRALI is Variable and Underreported

The reported incidence of TRALI is extremely variable and highly dependent on the inflammatory state and characteristics of the patient population studied.[20,21] Retrospective "look-back" studies suggest that TRALI is grossly under-recognized, so the incidence reported in studies utilizing passive surveillance underestimates the true incidence.[22,23] Only recently have prospective surveillance studies of transfused critically ill and operative patients recognized the alarming incidence of TRALI in the critically ill.[18,24–27] In the ICU, 37% to 44% of patients receive blood products, with the incidence rising to 85% in patients in the ICU for 7 days or longer.[1,28] Recent prospective observational trials demonstrate that 5% to 8% of all transfused patient admitted to a medical and surgical ICU develop TRALI. The incidence of TRALI is 2.4% in cardiac surgery and 1.3% in patient undergoing liver transplantation, but rises to 29% intransfused patients with chronic liver disease who are actively bleeding from varices.[24,27,29]

Evaluation of Risk for TRALI

When evaluating TRALI risk, two questions should be asked: what is the inflammatory state of the patient and what type and volume of planned blood component exposure is planned?

TRALI risk is highly dependent on the pretransfusion clinical state of the patient and the amount of exposure to blood components. In addition, different types of blood components carry different risks that are independent of the patient's clinical state. Therefore, both patient-specific and transfusion-specific factors need to be considered when determining the patient-specific risk versus benefit for each planned unit of transfused blood component.

TRALI is common in critically ill patients

The presence of multiple clinical risk factors for acute lung injury (ALI) increase the susceptibility to the subsequent development of TRALI.[30–32] Common risk factors for ALI include sepsis, trauma, aspiration, heavy alcohol use, mechanical ventilation, massive transfusion, and pneumonia.[14,24] More specifically, transfusion is an independent risk factor, in a dose-dependent manner, for the subsequent development of TRALI in patients with these preexisting ALI risk factors.[30,33–37] Consistent with the "two-event" mechanism, transfusion appears to act synergistically with other diagnoses that predispose patients to ALI. Two large prospective trials performed in the Unites States (n = 901) and Europe (n = 2024) demonstrate a TRALI incidence of 8% and 5% respectively. In these studies, sepsis and emergent surgery were strong independent risk factors for the development of TRALI. In addition, a cohort study of 225 patients admitted to an ICU due to gastrointestinal bleeding revealed a TRALI incidence of 29% in bleeding patients with chronic liver disease. In critically ill patients receiving massive transfusion the incidence of ALI is 21% to 45%, though these studies do not report the number of cases that were temporally related to transfusion (within 6 hours).[30,32,35] Collectively, these studies confirm the extraordinary high and variable incidence of TRALI in critically ill patients (**Fig. 1**).

TRALI can occur after the transfusion of any blood component

TRALI has been described after transfusion of most blood components including leukoreduced and non-leukoreduced PRBCs; plasma (fresh frozen, FP24, and thawed) from female multiparous, never pregnant, and male donors; platelets (apheresed, random donor or whole blood-derived); and a few case reports after

Transfusion-Related Acute Lung Injury (TRALI) in the critically ill

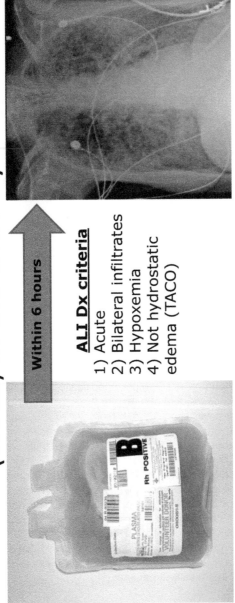

Within 6 hours

ALI Dx criteria
1) Acute
2) Bilateral infiltrates
3) Hypoxemia
4) Not hydrostatic edema (TACO)

- Associated most commonly with platelets and plasma
- Pre-existing inflammatory state increases risk (i.e. sepsis)
- TRALI is common in critically ill patients (5-8% of transfused ICU patients)
- Mortality of TRALI is 30-50% in ICU patients
- Antibody mediated (Anti-HLA I or II, anti-neutrophil) vs. non immune mediated

Fig. 1. Definition and risk factors for TRALI. TRALI is defined as ALI that develops within 6 hours of a transfused blood component and has a high mortality in ICU patients. TRALI is commonly due to plasma-containing blood components and is prevalent in ICU patients due to both antibody-mediated and non-antibody-mediated mechanisms.

transfusion of intravenous immunoglobulin (IVIG), cryoprecipitate, bone marrow stem cells, and transfused granulocytes.[38–41]

TRALI is more common after transfusion of plasma-containing blood products

Surveillance data are skewed toward severe cases of TRALI in which the diagnosis is clear and other possible etiologic risk factors for ALI are uncommonly present. It is known that antibody-mediated TRALI is more common in these instances, and as a result high-plasma–containing blood components such as platelets and plasma (fresh frozen or FP24) are more commonly implicated in these passive surveillance studies. A report from the Red Cross TRALI surveillance system implicates plasma as the etiologic agent in 75% of cases and 63% of deaths from TRALI.[42] An examination of reported TRALI fatalities to the United States Food and Drug Administration (FDA) implicated plasma in 50% of deaths reported.[43]

In critically ill patients, epidemiologic studies reporting an association between massive transfusion and the development of ALI failed to control for plasma that is universally administered as part of a massive transfusion protocol.[30–32] Plasma administration has emerged as an independent risk factor for TRALI in trauma, medical and surgical ICU populations.[18,33,37,44–46] In most of these studies, high-plasma containing blood products (fresh frozen plasma [FFP] and platelets), not PRBCs, were associated with TRALI.[18,33,44,46,47]

Management of TRALI

When TRALI is diagnosed, the management is similar to the management of ALI from other causes. This includes supportive care that entails optimization of mechanical ventilator parameters (low tidal volume) to avoid further injury to the lung while reducing pulmonary venous pressures with diuretics in patients without shock.[25,48] A restrictive transfusion strategy should be employed because transfusions in patients with existing ALI worsen outcomes.[35]

TRALI Prognosis

Mortality rates vary based on the patient population studied and are highly dependent on the relative health of the individual before the lung injury. In single-center studies TRALI-associated mortality was 6% to 13%.[19,49] National reporting systems likely overestimate the mortality rate in the general population owing to reporting bias for cases resulting in death, but underestimate the mortality risk in the ICU because these cases are rarely reported and tend to result in higher mortality rates. Hemovigilance data from Great Britain (SHOT), Quebec, and France reported TRALI mortality rates of 9%, 9.5%, and 15%, respectively.[50,51] In a nonselect group of critically ill patients the TRALI mortality is 41% to 53% while it is 92% in gastrointestinal bleeding patients with chronic liver disease. Cardiac surgery patients have an in-hospital TRALI mortality of 13% while the rate is 29% in liver transplantation.[29,52]

Prevention: Transfuse Safer Blood Components

Multiple attempts have been attempted to remove TRALI-causing mediators from stored blood components in an attempt to make the components we transfuse less likely to cause TRALI. These large-scale strategies have had variable effects and are discussed in the text that follows.

Leukoreduction and TRALI risk

Residual leukocytes contaminating stored PRBCs can theoretically potentiate TRALI by increasing the amount of lipids and inflammatory cytokines (IL-6. IL-8, TNF-α) that accumulate during storage.[53,54] These substances may act as a second hit when transfused into a patient with endothelial activation and/or primed neutrophils resulting in TRALI.[53,55,56] As a result of epidemiologic studies demonstrating an association between leukoreduction and improved outcomes, universal leukoreduction was adopted in most industrialized nations. Unfortunately, the majority of before and after studies as well as subsequent randomized controlled trials (RCTs) have failed to demonstrate a reduction in TRALI from leukoreduction.[57–59] Prestorage leukoreduction may reduce the accumulation of some of the biologically active mediators associated with storage, but does not significantly alter TRALI risk.

Age of blood and TRALI risk

Storage of RBCs results in a number of morphological and biochemical alterations known as the RBC storage lesion.[60] During routine storage of cellular components, a variety of neutrophil priming substances accumulate. Multiple epidemiologic studies have shown an association between increasing age of red blood cells and increased morbidity, mortality in trauma, medical and surgical ICU patients.[61–64] Age of blood was shown to be an independent risk factor for mortality in trauma after the institution of leukoreduction.[65,66] A recent small RCT demonstrated no difference in the changes in oxygenation in intubated patients after transfusion of 1 unit of fresh (4 day) versus old (27 day) PRBCs.[67] However, until the results from large multicenter clinical trials that are currently underway are available, the effect of storage duration on TRALI risk and outcome remains undefined.

Antibodies in high-plasma–containing blood components and TRALI risk

The majority of severe TRALI cases are associated with alloantibodies to leukocytes[6,19,42,49,68,69] High-plasma–containing blood components such as plasma (FFP or FP24) and platelets contain different types and concentrations of alloantibodies depending on the donor. In women reporting three or more pregnancies, 40% have presence of antibodies to either HLA class I, HLA class II, or granulocytes in donated plasma-containing components.[70] Several studies have demonstrated the clinical significance of female gender and multiparity of donor plasma and platelets on the recipient risk of developing antibody-mediated TRALI.[42,71,72] As a result, similar to the leukoreduction story, the majority of countries have transitioned to a male- and/or nonpregnant female–only donor policy for platelets and plasma. In addition, some countries have initiated antibody testing and other production techniques to reduce antibody contamination.[73,74] Fortunately, this blood banking strategy has reduced reported TRALI incidence and mortality in most before-and-after studies.[75–77]

In addition, a promising solvent/detergent process used for creating plasma removes antibodies and potentially other neutrophil-activating mediators. It is widely used in Europe, but has yet to receive FDA approval for use in the United States.[78] No TRALI cases have been reported to date using this process, and this plasma product has been demonstrated to be effective in reversing coagulopathic states.[76,78,79]

Prevention: Risk-Stratify Patients and Adjust Transfusion Strategy

The first step in preventing TRALI is educating practitioners regarding patient-specific risks while simultaneously enforcing the appropriate use of blood components. In the critically ill, one RCT has reported a significant decrease in the development of pulmonary edema by decreasing red blood cell transfusion thresholds.[80] In addition, transfusion of PRBCs rarely results in an improvement in oxygen utilization (the ultimate goal) at current PRBC transfusion thresholds (hemoglobin 8–10 mg/dL) in critically ill patients with sepsis.[25,81] Therefore the risk versus benefit of each unit of

RBC Transfusion in Critically ill
Risk vs. Benefit

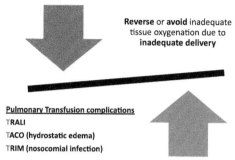

Reverse or avoid inadequate
tissue oxygenation due to
inadequate delivery

<u>Pulmonary Transfusion complications</u>
TRALI
TACO (hydrostatic edema)
TRIM (nosocomial infection)

Fig. 2. Weighing the risk vs. benefit of PRBC transfusion in the critically ill. Practitioners should weigh the pulmonary risks of PRBC transfusion against the physiologic benefit in critically ill patients. Reversing delivery dependent tissue hypoxia is a clear indication for PRBC transfusion. Other reasons for transfusion should be weighed against the most common and serious complications of PRBC transfusion in this patient population including TRALI, TACO, and TRIM.

PRBC transfused should be weighed heavily in the critically ill (**Fig. 2**). More restrictive plasma administration may have a potentially larger benefit because plasma is utilized inappropriately in 45% of hospitalized patients and 48% of critically ill patients.[82,83] In addition, current guideline use lacks level I evidence, and in many instances evidence suggests that plasma administration in bleeding patients or before minor procedures to correct coagulopathy lacks clinical benefit.[82,84–89] Ongoing clinical trials will be informative with regard to the risk-to-benefit ratio of preprocedural plasma in patients with coagulopathy.[90]

TACO

The FDA has reported TACO to be the second most common cause of transfusion-related mortality in the United States.[91,92] TACO is defined as pulmonary edema that develops in response to elevated pulmonary capillary hydrostatic pressures precipitated from the transfusion of blood components.[10] TACO usually develops within 2 hours of transfusion and can occur with any blood component because the volume, speed of transfusion, and oncotic properties of the transfused component are likely more important than type.[10] Initially, TACO is difficult to differentiate from TRALI because both lead to pulmonary edema and respiratory failure, but after a successful reduction in pulmonary capillary hydrostatic pressures with diuresis or dialysis pulmonary edema should resolve rapidly in patients with TACO. Other clues suggesting the diagnosis of TACO versus TRALI include peritransfusion hypertension, clinical clues to elevated left atrial hypertension, and lack of fever or leukopenia.[93,94] The use of brain natriuretic peptides to differentiate TRALI from TACO is controversial, but can be helpful at extremes.[95,96]

TACO is more common in critically ill patients, with an incidence of 6% in prospective studies, but the hospital mortality is significantly lower than TRALI at 8%.[97] The incidence is variable in other patient populations ranging from 1% to 8%.[47,93,98] TACO is also grossly under-recognized and underreported.[96,97] Risk factors include left ventricular dysfunction, plasma transfusion, and rate of transfusion.[91,92] Pretransfusion diuresis has not been demonstrated to be beneficial.[91] Clinical management includes reducing pulmonary capillary hydrostatic pressures with volume removal and/or a reduction in left ventricular afterload. Positive pressure ventilation is often needed to support the patient, which can also be beneficial in reducing pulmonary capillary hydrostatic pressures through left ventricular preload and afterload reduction.

Prevention of TACO requires recognition of at risk patients (left ventricular dysfunction and/or preexisting volume overload) and a determination that transfusion is truly indicated. Plasma is a common cause of TACO and often transfused in critically ill patients against guideline recommendation.[82,83] In high-risk patients in whom transfusion is clearly indicated, consider slowing the infusion rate and monitoring for hypoxemia.

TRIM

TRIM refers to the immunomodulatory effects of transfused blood components and the risk of subsequent infection to the transfused patient associated with this phenomenon. Early cohort studies demonstrated reductions in kidney transplant rejection and increased cancer recurrence associated with PRBC transfusion, leading to investigation of the immunomodulatory effect of PRBCs.[99,100] The mechanisms of immunomodulation are multifactorial, complex, and incompletely understood.[99,100] Since these early associations, multiple cohort studies have demonstrated a dose-dependent association between PRBC transfusion and the subsequent development of infection.[99,100] This association has yet to be confirmed in clinical trials, but the epidemiologic evidence is intriguing. Pulmonary complications result primarily from nosocomial pneumonia (including ventilator-associated pneumonia), which is the most deadly of the common infections associated with PRBC transfusion, but any infection causing severe sepsis can also lead to pulmonary complications from ALI and subsequent respiratory failure.[101–103]

Diagnosis can be inferred but not proven in patients developing a nosocomial or postoperative infection after they had been transfused PRBCs. Management is specific to the infectious source and includes antibiotics and source control. It is not possible to delineate the prognostic differences between infections developed in the setting of TRIM versus infections unrelated to transfusion because currently there is no method by which to differentiate etiology.[99] The patient population that bears the greatest risk are those undergoing cardiac surgery, as the effect of TRIM in other patient populations has been inconsistent in cohort studies.[104]

Currently it is debateable whether leukoreduction or age of blood reduces the infectious risk of PRBCs, but clinical trials are underway.[99,105–108] At present, the best strategy for prevention is to limit PRBC transfusion in critical care patients to clinical situations in which patients exhibit delivery-dependent tissue hypoxia or have the risk of developing this condition based on clinical course. Initiation of a restrictive PRBC transfusion protocol has demonstrated a reduced incidence of ventilator-associated pneumonia in one study.[109]

SUMMARY

In summary, the "terrible T's" of TRALI, TACO, and TRIM are all potentially fatal complications of blood transfusion. The mechanisms are multifactorial and complex, involving both transfusion-specific and patient-specific factors. Epidemiologic evidence suggests that these complications are more common in critically ill patients independent of the amount and type of transfused blood components transfused. Therefore, practitioners must be vigilant with respect to blood components in these patient populations. Transfused blood components should be administered only after careful consideration of the patient's unique risk of a transfusion complication versus the physiologic benefit of the planned transfused blood component. Blood components should be treated like pharmaceuticals, with continued refinement of the product in response to common and deadly side effects, and large multicenter trials performed to demonstrate efficacy. In the meantime, with regard to transfusion, less is often more.

REFERENCES

1. Corwin HL, Gettinger A, Pearl RG, et al. The CRIT Study: Anemia and blood transfusion in the critically ill—current clinical practice in the United States. Crit Care Med 2004;32(1):39–52.
2. Toy P, Popovsky MA, Abraham E, et al. Transfusion-related acute lung injury: definition and review. Crit Care Med 2005;33(4):721–6.
3. Keller-Stanislawski B, Lohmann A, Gunay S, et al. The German Haemovigilance System: reports of serious adverse transfusion reactions between 1997 and 2007. Transfus Med 2009;19(6):340–9.
4. Eder AF, Dy BA, Barton J, et al. The American Red Cross Hemovigilance Program: advancing the safety of blood donation and transfusion. Immunohematology 2009; 25(4):179–85.
5. Stainsby D, Jones H, Wells AW, et al. Adverse outcomes of blood transfusion in children: analysis of UK reports to the serious hazards of transfusion scheme 1996–2005. Br J Haematol 2008;141(1):73–9.
6. Win N, Massey E, Lucas G, et al. Ninety-six suspected transfusion related acute lung injury cases: investigation findings and clinical outcome. Hematology (Amsterdam) 2007;12(5):461–9.
7. van Stein D, Beckers EA, Sintnicolaas K, et al. Transfusion-related acute lung injury reports in the Netherlands: an observational study. Transfusion 2010;50(1):213–20.
8. Popovsky MA, Abel MD, Moore SB. Transfusion-related acute lung injury associated with passive transfer of antileukocyte antibodies. Am Rev Respir Dis 1983;128(1): 185–9.
9. Bernard GR, Artigas A, Brigham KL, et al. The American-European Consensus Conference on ARDS: definitions, mechanisms, relevant outcomes, and clinical trial coordination. Am J Respir Crit Care Med 1994;149(3 Pt 1):818–24.
10. Skeate RC, Eastlund T. Distinguishing between transfusion related acute lung injury and transfusion associated circulatory overload. Curr Opin Hematol 2007;14(6): 682–7.
11. Nakagawa M, Toy P. Acute and transient decrease in neutrophil count in transfusion-related acute lung injury: cases at one hospital. Transfusion 2004;44(12):1689–94.
12. Silliman CC, McLaughlin NJ. Transfusion-related acute lung injury. Blood Rev 2006;20(3):139–59.
13. Jy W, Ricci M, Shariatmadar S, et al. Microparticles in stored red blood cells as potential mediators of transfusion complications. Transfusion 2011;51(4):886–93.
14. Silliman CC, Fung YL, Ball JB, et al. Transfusion-related acute lung injury (TRALI): current concepts and misconceptions. Blood Rev 2009;23(6):245–55.
15. Looney MR, Gilliss BM, Matthay MA. Pathophysiology of transfusion-related acute lung injury. Curr Opin Hematol 2010;17(5):418–23.
16. Logdberg LE, Vikulina T, Zimring JC, et al. Animal models of transfusion-related acute lung injury. Transfus Med Rev 2009;23(1):13–24.

17. Fung YL, Silliman CC. The role of neutrophils in the pathogenesis of transfusion-related acute lung injury. Transfus Med Rev 2009;23(4):266–83.

18. Gajic O, Rana R, Winters JL, et al. Transfusion-related acute lung injury in the critically ill: prospective nested case-control study. Am J Respir Crit Care Med 2007;176(9):886–91.

19. Popovsky MA, Moore SB. Diagnostic and pathogenetic considerations in transfusion-related acute lung injury. Transfusion 1985;25(6):573–7.

20. Juffermans NP. Transfusion-related acute lung injury: emerging importance of host factors and implications for management. Expert Rev Hematol 2010;3(4):459–67.

21. Vlaar AP, Schultz MJ, Juffermans NP. Transfusion-related acute lung injury: a change of perspective. Neth J Med 2009;67(10):320–6.

22. Kopko PM, Marshall CS, MacKenzie MR, et al. Transfusion-related acute lung injury: report of a clinical look-back investigation. JAMA 2002;287(15):1968–71.

23. Kleinman S, Caulfield T, Chan P, et al. Toward an understanding of transfusion-related acute lung injury: statement of a consensus panel. Transfusion 2004;44(12): 1774–89.

24. Benson AB, Austin GL, Berg M, et al. Transfusion-related acute lung injury in ICU patients admitted with gastrointestinal bleeding. Intensive Care Med 2010;36(10): 1710–7.

25. Benson AB, Moss M, Silliman CC. Transfusion-related acute lung injury (TRALI): a clinical review with emphasis on the critically ill. Br J Haematol 2009;147(4):431–43.

26. Vlaar AP, Binnekade JM, Prins D, et al. Risk factors and outcome of transfusion-related acute lung injury in the critically ill: a nested case-control study. Crit Care Med 2010;38(3):771–8.

27. Vlaar AP, Hofstra JJ, Determann RM, et al. The incidence, risk factors and outcome of transfusion-related acute lung injury in a cohort of cardiac surgery patients: a prospective nested case control study. Blood 2011;117(16):4218–25.

28. Vincent JL, Baron JF, Reinhart K, et al. Anemia and blood transfusion in critically ill patients. JAMA 2002;288(12):1499–507.

29. Benson AB, Burton JR Jr, Austin GL, et al. Differential effects of plasma and red blood cell transfusions on acute lung injury and infection risk following liver transplantation. Liver Transpl 2011;17(2):149–58.

30. Hudson LD, Milberg JA, Anardi D, et al. Clinical risks for development of the acute respiratory distress syndrome. Am J Respir Crit Care Med 1995;151(2 Pt 1):293–301.

31. Fowler AA, Hamman RF, Good JT, et al. Adult respiratory distress syndrome: risk with common predispositions. Ann Intern Med 1983;98(5 Pt 1):593–7.

32. Pepe PE, Potkin RT, Reus DH, et al. Clinical predictors of the adult respiratory distress syndrome. Am J Surg 1982;144(1):124–30.

33. Gajic O, Rana R, Mendez JL, et al. Acute lung injury after blood transfusion in mechanically ventilated patients. Transfusion 2004;44(10):1468–74.

34. Croce MA, Tolley EA, Claridge JA, et al. Transfusions result in pulmonary morbidity and death after a moderate degree of injury. J Trauma 2005;59(1):19–23.

35. Gong MN, Thompson BT, Williams P, et al. Clinical predictors of and mortality in acute respiratory distress syndrome: potential role of red cell transfusion. Crit Care Med 2005;33(6):1191–8.

36. Silverboard H, Aisiku I, Martin GS, et al. The role of acute blood transfusion in the development of acute respiratory distress syndrome in patients with severe trauma. J Trauma 2005;59(3):717–23.

37. Chaiwat O, Lang JD, Vavilala MS, et al. Early packed red blood cell transfusion and acute respiratory distress syndrome after trauma. Anesthesiology 2009; 110(2):351–60.
38. Rizk A, Gorson KC, Kenney L, et al. Transfusion-related acute lung injury after the infusion of IVIG. Transfusion 2001;41(2):264–8.
39. Sachs UJ, Bux J. TRALI after the transfusion of cross-match-positive granulocytes. Transfusion 2003;43(12):1683–6.
40. Reese EP Jr, McCullough JJ, Craddock PR. An adverse pulmonary reaction to cryoprecipitate in a hemophiliac. Transfusion 1975;15(6):583–8.
41. Urahama N, Tanosaki R, Masahiro K, et al. TRALI after the infusion of marrow cells in a patient with acute lymphoblastic leukemia. Transfusion 2003;43(11):1553–7.
42. Eder AF, Herron R, Strupp A, et al. Transfusion-related acute lung injury surveillance (2003–2005) and the potential impact of the selective use of plasma from male donors in the American Red Cross. Transfusion 2007;47(4):599–607.
43. Holness L, Knippen MA, Simmons L, et al. Fatalities caused by TRALI. Transfus Med Rev 2004;18(3):184–8.
44. Khan H, Belsher J, Yilmaz M, et al. Fresh-frozen plasma and platelet transfusions are associated with development of acute lung injury in critically ill medical patients. Chest 2007;131(5):1308–14.
45. Gajic O, Yilmaz M, Iscimen R, et al. Transfusion from male-only versus female donors in critically ill recipients of high plasma volume components. Crit Care Med 2007; 35(7):1645–8.
46. Sadis C, Dubois MJ, Melot C, et al. Are multiple blood transfusions really a cause of acute respiratory distress syndrome? Eur J Anaesthesiol 2007;24(4):355–61.
47. Rana R, Fernandez-Perez ER, Khan SA, et al. Transfusion-related acute lung injury and pulmonary edema in critically ill patients: a retrospective study. Transfusion 2006;46(9):1478–83.
48. Wheeler AP, Bernard GR. Acute lung injury and the acute respiratory distress syndrome: a clinical review. Lancet 2007;369(9572):1553–64.
49. Popovsky MA, Haley NR. Further characterization of transfusion-related acute lung injury: demographics, clinical and laboratory features, and morbidity. Immunohematol Am Red Cross 2000;16(4):157–9.
50. Bux J. Transfusion-related acute lung injury (TRALI): a serious adverse event of blood transfusion. Vox Sang 2005;89(1):1–10.
51. Rebibo D, Hauser L, Slimani A, et al. The French haemovigilance system: organization and results for 2003. Transfus Apher Sci 2004;31(2):145–53.
52. Vlaar AP, Cornet AD, Hofstra JJ, et al. The effect of blood transfusion on pulmonary permeability in cardiac surgery patients: a prospective multicenter cohort study. Transfusion 2011;52(1):82–90.
53. Silliman CC, Paterson AJ, Dickey WO, et al. The association of biologically active lipids with the development of transfusion-related acute lung injury: a retrospective study. Transfusion 1997;37(7):719–26.
54. Kristiansson M, Soop M, Saraste L, et al. Cytokines in stored red blood cell concentrates: promoters of systemic inflammation and simulators of acute transfusion reactions? Acta Anaesthesiol Scand 1996;40(4):496–501.
55. Luk CS, Gray-Statchuk LA, Cepinkas G, et al. WBC reduction reduces storage-associated RBC adhesion to human vascular endothelial cells under conditions of continuous flow in vitro. Transfusion 2003;43(2):151–6.
56. Silliman CC, Voelkel NF, Allard JD, et al. Plasma and lipids from stored packed red blood cells cause acute lung injury in an animal model. J Clin Invest 1998;101(7): 1458–67.

57. Hebert PC, Fergusson D, Blajchman MA, et al. Clinical outcomes following institution of the Canadian universal leukoreduction program for red blood cell transfusions. JAMA 2003;289(15):1941–9.

58. Watkins TR, Rubenfeld GD, Martin TR, et al. Effects of leukoreduced blood on acute lung injury after trauma: a randomized controlled trial. Crit Care Med 2008;36(5): 1493–9.

59. Dzik WH, Anderson JK, O'Neill EM, et al. A prospective, randomized clinical trial of universal WBC reduction. Transfusion 2002;42(9):1114–22.

60. Kim-Shapiro DB, Lee J, Gladwin MT. Storage lesion: role of red blood cell break-down. Transfusion 2011;51(4):844–51.

61. Basran S, Frumento RJ, Cohen A, et al. The association between duration of storage of transfused red blood cells and morbidity and mortality after reoperative cardiac surgery. Anesth Analg 2006;103(1):15–20.

62. Purdy FR, Tweeddale MG, Merrick PM. Association of mortality with age of blood transfused in septic ICU patients. Can J Anaesth (J Can d'Anesth) 1997;44(12): 1256–61.

63. Zallen G, Offner PJ, Moore EE, et al. Age of transfused blood is an independent risk factor for postinjury multiple organ failure. Am J Surg 1999;178(6):570–2.

64. Koch CG, Li L, Sessler DI, et al. Duration of red-cell storage and complications after cardiac surgery. N Engl J Med 2008;358(12):1229–39.

65. Weinberg JA, McGwin G Jr, Griffin RL, et al. Age of transfused blood: an indepen-dent predictor of mortality despite universal leukoreduction. J Trauma 2008;65(2): 279–82.

66. Weinberg JA, McGwin G Jr, Marques MB, et al. Transfusions in the less severely injured: does age of transfused blood affect outcomes? J Trauma 2008;65(4): 794–8.

67. Kor DJ, Kashyap R, Weiskopf RB, et al. Fresh red blood cell transfusion and short-term pulmonary, immunologic, and coagulation status: a randomized clinical trial. Am J Respir Crit Care Med 2012;185(8):842–50.

68. Kopko PM, Popovsky MA, MacKenzie MR, et al. HLA class II antibodies in transfu-sion-related acute lung injury. Transfusion 2001;41(10):1244–8.

69. Lydaki E, Bolonaki E, Nikoloudi E, et al. HLA class II antibodies in transfusion-related acute lung injury (TRALI): a case report. Transfus Apher Sci 2005;33(2):107–11.

70. Sachs UJ, Link E, Hofmann C, et al. Screening of multiparous women to avoid transfusion-related acute lung injury: a single centre experience. Transfus Med (Oxford) 2008;18(6):348–54.

71. Chapman CE, Stainsby D, Jones H, et al. Ten years of hemovigilance reports of transfusion-related acute lung injury in the United Kingdom and the impact of preferential use of male donor plasma. Transfusion 2009;49(3):440–52.

72. Vlaar AP, Binnekade JM, Schultz MJ, et al. Preventing TRALI: ladies first, what follows? Crit Care Med 2008;36(12):3283–4 [author reply: 3284].

73. Lin Y, Saw CL, Hannach B, et al. Transfusion-related acute lung injury prevention measures and their impact at Canadian Blood Services. Transfusion 2011;52(3): 567–74.

74. Lucas G, Win N, Calvert A, et al. Reducing the incidence of TRALI in the UK: the results of screening for donor leucocyte antibodies and the development of national guidelines. Vox Sang 2011;103(1):10–7.

75. Wright SE, Snowden CP, Athey SC, et al. Acute lung injury after ruptured abdominal aortic aneurysm repair: the effect of excluding donations from females from the production of fresh frozen plasma. Crit Care Med 2008;36(6):1796–802.

76. Ozier Y, Muller JY, Mertes PM, et al. Transfusion-related acute lung injury: reports to the French Hemovigilance Network 2007 through 2008. Transfusion 2011;51(10): 2102–10.
77. Wiersum-Osselton JC, Middelburg RA, Beckers EA, et al. Male-only fresh-frozen plasma for transfusion-related acute lung injury prevention: before-and-after comparative cohort study. Transfusion 2011;51(6):1278–83.
78. Hellstern P, Solheim BG. The use of solvent/detergent treatment in pathogen reduction of plasma. Transfus Med Hemother 2011;38(1):65–70.
79. Carvalho MC, Rodrigues AG, Conceicao LM, et al. Prothrombin complex concentrate (Octaplex): a Portuguese experience in 1152 patients. Blood Coagul Fibrinolysis 2012;23(3):222–8.
80. Hebert PC, Wells G, Blajchman MA, et al for Transfusion Requirements in Critical Care Investigators, Canadian Critical Care Trials Group. A multicenter, randomized, controlled clinical trial of transfusion requirements in critical care. N Engl J Med 1999;340(6):409–17.
81. Marik PE, Corwin HL. Acute lung injury following blood transfusion: expanding the definition. Crit Care Med 2008;36(11):3080–4.
82. Lauzier F, Cook D, Griffith L, et al. Fresh frozen plasma transfusion in critically ill patients. Crit Care Med 2007;35(7):1655–9.
83. Luk C, Eckert KM, Barr RM, et al. Prospective audit of the use of fresh-frozen plasma, based on Canadian Medical Association transfusion guidelines. CMAJ 2002;166(12):1539–40.
84. Kozek-Langenecker S, Sorensen B, Hess J, et al. Clinical effectiveness of fresh frozen plasma compared with fibrinogen concentrate: a systematic review. Crit Care 2011;15(5):R239.
85. Verghese SG. Elective fresh frozen plasma in the critically ill: what is the evidence? Crit Care Resusc 2008;10(3):264–8.
86. Dara SI, Rana R, Afessa B, et al. Fresh frozen plasma transfusion in critically ill medical patients with coagulopathy. Crit Care Med 2005;33(11):2667–71.
87. Tripodi A. Tests of coagulation in liver disease. Clin Liver Dis 2009;13(1):55–61.
88. Wallis JP, Dzik S. Is fresh frozen plasma overtransfused in the United States? Transfusion 2004;44(11):1674–5.
89. Holland L, Sarode R. Should plasma be transfused prophylactically before invasive procedures? Curr Opin Hematol 2006;13(6):447–51.
90. Muller MC, de Jonge E, Arbous MS, et al. Transfusion of fresh frozen plasma in non-bleeding ICU patients—TOPIC TRIAL: study protocol for a randomized controlled trial. Trials 2011;12(1):266.
91. Li G, Rachmale S, Kojicic M, et al. Incidence and transfusion risk factors for transfusion-associated circulatory overload among medical intensive care unit patients. Transfusion 2011;51(2):338–43.
92. Narick C, Triulzi DJ, Yazer MH. Transfusion-associated circulatory overload after plasma transfusion. Transfusion 2012;52(1):160–5.
93. Gajic O, Gropper MA, Hubmayr RD. Pulmonary edema after transfusion: how to differentiate transfusion-associated circulatory overload from transfusion-related acute lung injury. Crit Care Med 2006;34(5 Suppl):S109–13.
94. Popovsky MA. Pulmonary consequences of transfusion: TRALI and TACO. Transfus Apher Sci 2006;34(3):243–4.
95. Tobian AA, Sokoll LJ, Tisch DJ, et al. N-terminal pro-brain natriuretic peptide is a useful diagnostic marker for transfusion-associated circulatory overload. Transfusion 2008;48(6):1143–50.

96. Li G, Daniels CE, Kojicic M, et al. The accuracy of natriuretic peptides (brain natriuretic peptide and N-terminal pro-brain natriuretic) in the differentiation between transfusion-related acute lung injury and transfusion-related circulatory overload in the critically ill. Transfusion 2009;49(1):13–20.

97. Li G, Kojicic M, Reriani MK, et al. Long-term survival and quality of life after transfusion-associated pulmonary edema in critically ill medical patients. Chest 2010;137(4):783–9.

98. Popovsky MA, Audet AM, Andrzejewski C Jr. Transfusion-associated circulatory overload in orthopedic surgery patients: a multi-institutional study. Immunohematology 1996;12(2):87–9.

99. Vamvakas EC, Blajchman MA. Transfusion-related immunomodulation (TRIM): an update. Blood Rev 2007;21(6):327–48.

100. Buddeberg F, Schimmer BB, Spahn DR. Transfusion-transmissible infections and transfusion-related immunomodulation. Best Pract Res Clin Anaesthesiol 2008; 22(3):503–17.

101. Shorr AF, Duh MS, Kelly KM, et al. Red blood cell transfusion and ventilator-associated pneumonia: a potential link? Crit Care Med 2004;32(3):666–74.

102. Taylor RW, Manganaro L, O'Brien J, et al. Impact of allogenic packed red blood cell transfusion on nosocomial infection rates in the critically ill patient. Crit Care Med 2002;30(10):2249–54.

103. Gunst MA, Minei JP. Transfusion of blood products and nosocomial infection in surgical patients. Curr Opin Crit Care 2007;13(4):428–32.

104. Bilgin YM, Brand A. Transfusion-related immunomodulation: a second hit in an inflammatory cascade? Vox Sang 2008;95(4):261–71.

105. Sparrow RL. Red blood cell storage and transfusion-related immunomodulation. Blood Transfus 2010;8(Suppl 3):s26–30.

106. Parker RI. Transfusion-related immunomodulation: how much of it is due to white cells? Pediatr Crit Care Med 2011;12(5):593–4.

107. Yepes D, Gil B, Hernandez O, et al. Ventilator associated pneumonia and transfusion: is there really an association? (the NAVTRA study). BMC Pulm Med 2006;6:18.

108. Vamvakas EC, Carven JH. Transfusion and postoperative pneumonia in coronary artery bypass graft surgery: effect of the length of storage of transfused red cells. Transfusion 1999;39(7):701–10.

109. Yepes D, Gil B. Anemia management program reduces transfusion volumes, incidence of ventilator-associated pneumonia, and cost in trauma patients. J Trauma 2007;62(4):1065.

Management of COPD Patients in the Intensive Care Unit

Paula McCauley, DNP APRN ACNP-BC[a,b,*], Debapriya Datta, MD, FCCP[c]

KEYWORDS

- Chronic obstructive pulmonary disease • Ventilation • Noninvasive ventilation
- Pulmonary rehabilitation • Palliative care

KEY POINTS

- Chronic obstructive pulmonary disease (COPD) is a disease characterized by expiratory airflow limitation that is not fully reversible.
- Acute respiratory failure, altered mental status, and hemodynamic instability associated with acute exacerbations of COPD are commonly encountered and require careful management in the intensive care unit setting.
- Noninvasive and invasive ventilator support in conjunction with pharmacotherapy can be lifesaving.

INTRODUCTION

Chronic obstructive pulmonary disease (COPD) is a disease characterized by progressive, persistent, expiratory airflow limitation that is not fully reversible.[1,2] In the United States, COPD annually accounts for $29.5 billion in direct health care costs,[3] 750,000 hospitalizations, and 1.5 million emergency visits.[4] Globally it is now ranked as the fifth leading cause of death.[1,3,4] COPD is generally described as a progressive disease; however, there is considerable variability among patients.[5] Exacerbations are often the cause of morbidity and mortality in COPD patients.[1,2,6] An exacerbation of COPD is characterized by an acute worsening of a patient's respiratory symptoms that results in change in treatment and increased utilization of health care resources. Most exacerbations can be managed in the outpatient setting; however, patients with more severe underlying disease or exacerbation may require hospitalization. Acute

The authors have nothing to disclose.
[a] University of Connecticut School of Nursing, 231 Glenbrook Road, Unit 2026, Storrs, CT 06269, USA; [b] Critical Care, Surgery Division, University of Connecticut Health Center, 263 Farmington Avenue, Farmington, CT 06030, USA; [c] Division of Pulmonary, Critical Care and Sleep Medicine, University of Connecticut Health Center, 263 Farmington Avenue, Farmington, CT 06030, USA
* University of Connecticut School of Nursing, 231 Glenbrook Road, Unit 2026, Storrs, CT 06269-2026.
E-mail address: paula.mccauley@uconn.edu

exacerbations in patients with moderate to severe COPD can cause respiratory failure and a possible need for ventilatory support. Patients with acute exacerbation of COPD causing acute respiratory failure with severe hypoxia or persistent or severe respiratory acidosis, altered mental status, or hemodynamic instability require admission to an intensive care unit (ICU) for management.

The objective of this review is to briefly elucidate the clinical features of COPD and management of exacerbations and provide a detailed description of management of COPD in the ICU, including indications for admission to ICU and treatment of acute respiratory failure in COPD in the ICU, in terms of pharmacologic and ventilatory therapy. Advance care planning, rehabilitation, and palliative care are necessary components for comprehensive critical care of these patients.

CLINICAL FEATURES OF COPD

COPD is a preventable and treatable disease. COPD is preventable because the majority of cases are the result of cigarette smoking. It is treatable because maintenance with long-term bronchodilators has been shown to improve lung function and reduce the frequency of exacerbations. The expiratory airflow limitation that characterizes COPD is usually progressive and is associated with an abnormal inflammatory response of the lungs to noxious particles or gases, mainly cigarette smoking. Diagnosis of COPD should be considered in any patient with chronic cough or sputum production, dyspnea, and/or a history of exposure to risk factors for the disease. Physical examination in a patient with COPD may be normal, especially in mild stages of the disease. Diminished breath sounds with prolonged expiratory phase (>4 seconds) are usually found in patients with symptomatic disease. Rhonchi and wheezes indicate bronchospasm and may be heard on lung auscultation but are not consistent findings. They are more likely to be heard with exacerbations. In severe disease, characteristic physical signs such as increased accessory muscle use, pursed lip breathing to facilitate exhalation, and signs of pulmonary hypertension and right heart failure may be apparent. Although COPD affects the lungs, it also produces significant extrapulmonary effects such as cor pulmonale, osteoporosis, skeletal muscle dysfunction, weight loss, and depression. Systemic co-morbidities of COPD include myocardial infarction, congestive heart failure (CHF), arrhythmia, and venous thromboembolism (VTE).[7]

The diagnosis of COPD is made by spirometry, demonstrating the presence of airflow limitation that is not fully reversible with a post-bronchodilator FEV1/FVC (forced expiratory volume in 1 second over the forced vital capacity) ratio less than 0.70.[1,2] Diffusion capacity may be decreased in COPD due to destruction of alveoli and loss of alveolar capillary basement membrane. Due to loss of elastic recoil of the lung, hyperinflation occurs with an increase in total lung capacity (TLC). Increase in residual volume (RV) may also be seen and reflects air trapping. Spirometric classification is useful in guiding care and monitoring the progression of disease.

While the presence of airway obstruction is determined by a ratio of FEV_1 to forced vital capacity of less than 0.07, the severity of COPD is based on the post-bronchodilator FEV_1 (forced expiratory volume in 1 second) as follows[1,2,8]:

- Stage 1: Mild—FEV_1/FVC < 0.7; FEV_1 ≥ 80% predicted
- Stage 2: Moderate—FEV_1/FVC < 0.7; FEV_1 ≥ 50% predicted to ≤ 80% predicted
- Stage 3: Severe—FEV_1/FVC < 0.7; FEV_1 ≥ 30% predicted to ≤ 50% predicted
- Stage 4: Very severe—FEV_1/FVC < 0.7; FEV_1 < 30% predicted.

In addition to FEV_1, exercise capacity and dyspnea have proven to be useful in predicting outcomes such as survival in large cohorts of patients. Celli and

---

Box 1
Treatment modalities of stable COPD

- Bronchodilators
  (a) Short-acting bronchodilators such as albuterol, ipratropium
  (b) Long-acting bronchodilators such as salmeterol, tiotropium
- Inhaled corticosteroids
- Supplemental oxygen therapy if hypoxia present
- Pulmonary rehabilitation

---

colleagues[9] reported on four factors: the body mass index (B) obtained by dividing the weight (in kg) over the square of the height (in m^2); the degree of airflow obstruction (O) measured by FEV_1; dyspnea (D) measured by the Modified Medical Research Council (MMRC) Scale; and exercise capacity (E), measured by the 6-minute–walk test predictive of mortality. These variables were used to generate the BODE index, a multidimensional 10-point scale, based on points ranging from 0 to 3 for severity of each variable. This study established that higher scores indicate a higher risk of death in patients with COPD. This index has been found to be a much better predictor of mortality than FEV_1 alone. BMI values less than $21 \text{ kg} \cdot m^{-2}$ are also associated with increased mortality.

MANAGEMENT OF STABLE COPD

Treatment of COPD is aimed at (1) improving airflow obstruction, (2) providing symptomatic relief, (3) modifying or preventing exacerbations, and (4) altering disease progression. Treatment modalities of stable COPD are shown in **Box 1**.

Bronchodilators are used in COPD for prevention of symptoms (maintenance therapy) as well as to acutely relieve symptoms (rescue inhalers). Bronchodilators act by altering the bronchial smooth muscle tone and reducing dynamic hyperinflation (air trapping) at rest and with exertion. Maintenance medications include long-acting β_2-agonists such as salmeterol and formoterol and long-acting anticholinergics such as tiotropium for prevention of symptoms. Short-acting bronchodilators are used for the acute relief of symptoms, including the β_2-agonist albuterol and anticholinergics such as ipratropium. The preferred mode of administration of these bronchodilators is by metered dose inhaler (MDI) or dry powder inhaler (DPI).[1,2]

Inhaled corticosteroids provide anti-inflammatory therapy. Because patients with COPD often have an underlying inflammatory process, inhaled corticosteroids are sometimes used to stabilize the inflammatory process as well as to reduce the frequency of exacerbations.

Supplemental oxygen therapy is indicated in patients with COPD with resting P_aO_2 of 55 mm Hg or lower on room air or P_aO_2 of 56 mm Hg or greater and 59 mm Hg or lower in conjunction with cor pulmonale or erythocytocis (hematocrit >55%).[1,2] A decrease in oxygen saturation (SaO_2) to less than 88% with normal walking is an indication for supplemental O_2 with activity.[1] Pulmonary rehabilitation has become an established mode of treatment to improve functional capacity and reduce symptoms of dyspnea in patients with COPD.[1,2]

Acute Exacerbations of COPD

An exacerbation of COPD is an "event in the natural course of the disease characterized by a change in the patient's baseline dyspnea, cough and/or sputum that is beyond normal day-to-day variations."[1(p40)] The variability is sufficient to warrant a change in management. Though the majority of exacerbations can be managed in an outpatient setting, despite aggressive medical treatment, approximately one third of patients discharged from the emergency department with acute exacerbations have a recurrence within 14 days,[1,10] and 17% relapse and require hospitalization.[11] Mortality for exacerbations requiring hospitalizations are approximately 2%, increasing to 20% if the patient requires mechanical ventilation.[12] In addition, although most exacerbations are related to a bacterial or viral infection, the causes of a third of cases are never identified. The cost of an exacerbation is substantial. In 2006, more than a million hospitalizations occurred at a cost of $11.9 billion.[12] The best predictor of an exacerbation is a history of a prior exacerbation, irrespective of severity of COPD.[13]

Patients with an exacerbation of COPD require hospitalization in the following settings[1]:

1. Frequent exacerbations
2. Worsening hypoxemia or hypercapnia
3. Changes in mental status
4. Concomitant presence of any of these comorbid conditions: CHF, cardiac arrhythmia, diabetes mellitus, renal or liver failure, and pneumonia
5. Inadequate response to outpatient management
6. Inability of the patient to be cared for and/or to care for her- or himself at home
7. Advancing age.

Treatment for a hospitalized patient with acute exacerbation of COPD includes bronchodilator therapy with short-acting β_2-agonist (albuterol, salbutamol) and/or ipratropium, administered via spacer or nebulizer as needed.[14,15] Corticosteroids therapy should be started in these patients: oral prednisone 30 to 40 mg/day or intravenous equivalent dose if the patient cannot tolerate oral intake with subsequent transition to oral. Steroids should be tapered over 10 to 14 days.[16,17] Supplemental oxygen should be administered for O_2 saturation of less than 90%. Antibiotics[18,19] should be initiated in patients who have a change in their sputum characteristics (purulence and/or increased volume) or obvious radiographic or microbiological evidence of respiratory tract infection. Choice of antibiotic should be based on local bacteria resistance patterns. Per the American Thoracic Society/European Respiratory Society (ATS/ERS) guidelines, macrolides, amoxicillin/clavulanate, or respiratory fluoroquinolones may be options for use in an acute exacerbation.[1,2] If infection with *Pseudomonas* and/or other Enterobacteriaceae species is suspected, combination therapy should be considered.

MANAGEMENT OF COPD PATIENTS IN THE ICU

The need for admission to an ICU is based on the severity of respiratory failure. Patients with severe exacerbations of COPD may be admitted to intermediate care units if skilled and experienced personnel and equipment are available to provide appropriate care and manage acute respiratory failure successfully. The indications for admission to an ICU or a special respiratory care unit are summarized in **Box 2**.[1]

COPD negatively impacts long-term survival. Specific factors, including advanced age and cardiovascular, neurologic, or renal dysfunction increase

---

Box 2

Indications for ICU admission

- Acute respiratory failure, actual or impending
- Hemodynamic instability
- Altered mental status/inability to protect airways

---

morbidity and mortality. Length of stay and invasive mechanical ventilation are also associated with an increase in mortality.[20] Treatment of patients in a special unit or ICU is similar to treatment of hospitalized non-ICU patients in terms of pharmacologic therapy with nebulized bronchodilators, corticosteroids, and antibiotics. Patients with respiratory failure require ventilatory support, which may be either invasive or noninvasive.

Ventilatory Support of COPD Patients

Mechanical ventilation in COPD patients in the ICU aims at providing supportive therapy while underlying acute exacerbation of COPD and the consequent acute respiratory failure are reversed with medical therapy.[21,22] Mechanical ventilation should be instituted when, despite appropriate medical therapy and oxygen administration, there is no significant improvement in moderate to severe respiratory acidosis (pH < 7.36) and the work of breathing.

Modes of Mechanical Ventilation

Mechanical ventilation can be delivered through an endotracheal or tracheostomy tube (invasive mechanical ventilation) or through the use of a mask, without the use of an endotracheal tube (noninvasive mechanical ventilation), which is also known as noninvasive positive pressure ventilation (NPPV).

NPPV

NPPV represents a major advancement in the treatment of acute exacerbations of COPD in the ICU. NPPV has resulted in lesser number of intubations and invasive mechanical ventilation being performed, and has also significantly reduced mortality for severe COPD exacerbations. NPPV is by far the most commonly used mode of providing noninvasive ventilation.[22,23] Commonly used modes of NPPV include continuous positive airway pressure (CPAP) plus pressure support ventilation (PSV) or bilevel positive airway pressure (BIPAP).

NPPV should be administered to patients with exacerbations when, after optimal medical therapy and oxygenation, respiratory acidosis (pH <7.36) and or respiratory distress persists. For pH less than 7.30, NPPV should be delivered under controlled environments such as intermediate care units or high-dependency respiratory units (in institutions where they exist) where close monitoring of patients can be performed, with facilities for rapid endotracheal intubation and institution of conventional mechanical ventilation promptly available. If pH is less than 7.25, NPPV should be administered in the ICU with intubation being readily available. Settings of BIPAP with inspiratory positive airway pressure (IPAP) of 10 to 15 and expiratory positive airway pressure (EPAP) of 4 to 6 or the combination of pressure support (PS) of 10 to 15 cm H_2O and CPAP of 4 to 8 cm H_2O provides

---

Box 3
Contraindications to NPPV

- Respiratory or cardiac arrest
- Hemodynamic instability (hypotension, arrhythmias)
- Myocardial infarction
- Impaired mental status, inability to cooperate
- Excessive airway secretions
- Inability to use mask due to recent facial surgery or trauma
- Upper airway obstruction

---

an effective mode of NPPV. Contraindications to the use of NPPV are shown in **Box 3.** Patients with contraindications to NPPV or failing therapy with NPPV should be intubated and placed on invasive mechanical ventilation.

Several controlled trials have shown that NPPV is effective in the treatment of acute respiratory failure with COPD exacerbation.[24] In addition to randomized clinical trials, high-quality meta-analyses have shown that NPPV is very effective and safe in exacerbations of COPD[25] with respiratory acidosis.[26] The patients most likely to benefit from NPPV are those with elevated arterial carbon dioxide, who are able to cooperate with the caregivers and with no coexisting comorbid problems such as sepsis, severe pneumonia, cardiovascular instability, and arrhythmias.

In patients with severe respiratory acidosis (pH <7.25), NPPV may be as effective as conventional mechanical ventilation to reverse acute respiratory failure due to COPD.[27,28] One-year mortality was reported to be lower in patients receiving NPPV for exacerbations of COPD, compared to both patients receiving optimal medical therapy alone[29] and those receiving conventional mechanical ventilation.[30] NPPV should be considered as the first-line intervention, in addition to optimal medical therapy, for the management of patients with respiratory failure due to exacerbation of COPD.[25] In the first few hours of initiation, NPPV requires the same level of assistance as conventional mechanical ventilation.

Studies have shown that NPPV is highly cost effective in exacerbation of COPD complicated by acute respiratory failure.[31] In patients on invasive ventilation, with weaning failure, NPPV can be used successfully for weaning.[32,33] Factors associated with successful outcome with NPPV include younger age, ability to cooperate, lower acuity of illness, experienced caregivers, and availability of resources for monitoring.[1,2]

Invasive ventilation/conventional mechanical ventilation

Intubation and institution of conventional mechanical ventilation should be considered in patients in the following situations:

1. When NPPV fails: worsening of arterial blood gases and or pH in 1–2 h; lack of improvement in arterial blood gases and/or pH after 4 h
2. Severe respiratory acidosis (pH <7.25) despite use of NPPV
3. Life-threatening hypoxia (P_aO_2 <50 mm Hg)
4. Severe respiratory distress with increased work of breathing and respiratory rate greater than 35 breaths/min

5. Hemodynamic instability
6. When NPPV is contraindicated, not tolerated, or in cases of impending respiratory arrest.

Usually patients with COPD with acute respiratory failure are started on assist control (AC) mode of ventilation. Low tidal volumes of 6 mL/kg as are used in acute respiratory distress syndrome (ARDS) patients are not mandatory but may be required to reduce auto positive end-expiratory pressure (PEEP). Initial ventilator settings in these patients may be AC at a rate of 10 to 12 breaths/min, tidal volume of 8 to 10 mL/kg of predicted body weight, F_iO_2 as required to maintain oxygen saturation at greater than 90% and PEEP of 0 to 5. Based on adequacy of oxygenation and ventilation as evidenced on arterial blood gas as well as patients response to mechanical ventilation, ventilator parameters may be further modified. It is important to remember that the goal of ventilation is to achieve po_2 of 60 mm Hg or greater and a pco_2 that is the patient's baseline value with a normal or near normal pH. Patients with COPD may have chronic hypercapnia and should not be ventilated to achieve a normal pco_2.[1]

Mechanical ventilation in patients with COPD can present certain challenges. Due to increased airway resistance and air trapping in these patients, patients are prone to develop intrinsic PEEP or auto PEEP.[30] Auto PEEP can have adverse hemodynamic consequences that can be life-threatening. To reduce auto PEEP, exhalation time should be prolonged by either reducing rate or tidal volume and/or applying extrinsic PEEP. Aggressive inhaled bronchodilator therapy should be administered to reduce airway resistance. Ventilator dysynchrony should be prevented with adequate sedation. In some cases, neuromuscular blockade may be required to counter patient–ventilator dysynchrony.

If respiratory acidosis persists on AC with pH less than 7.30, minute ventilation should be increased. If the patient's plateau pressure (P_{pl}) is greater than 30 cm H_2O, tidal volume may be increased. If P_{pl} is greater than 30 cm H_2O, respiratory rate may be increased or mild to moderate elevated levels of CO_2 with consequent respiratory acidosis may be tolerated (permissive hypercapnia). An important point to remember is that ventilation in respiratory failure in COPD should be directed at normalizing the pH and not the pco_2.[34]

Medical therapy of the exacerbation of COPD, including bronchodilators, systemic steroids, and antibiotics should continue concomitantly. Patients require sedation, nutritional support, and gastrointestinal and deep venous thrombosis prophylaxis while on ventilator support. Because of the administration of systemic steroids, they are likely to develop hyperglycemia. Blood glucose levels should be periodically checked and corrected with insulin therapy to maintain blood glucose levels of less than 180 g/dL. All metabolic and electrolyte derangements should be corrected if present. Daily sedation holidays are also important, as in any critically ill patient in the ICU, to optimize sedation and reduce the risk of oversedation causing increased duration of ventilator support.

Once patients show clinical improvement, usually in 48 to 72 hours, spontaneous breathing trials should be attempted. Weaning trial should be performed once the patient's F_iO_2 requirement is 50% or less, the patient is hemodynamically stable, awake enough to protect his or her airway, and does not have copious secretions requiring frequent pulmonary toilet. On pressure support weaning mode, which is the more commonly used spontaneous breathing trial (SBT) in ICUs, lung mechanics and extubation parameters are determined. If these are satisfactory (**Box 4**), the patient can be extubated. In patients who fail weaning,

---

Box 4
Extubation parameters for patients with COPD with acute respiratory failure

1. Respiratory rate $\leq$ 30 breaths/min

2. Spontaneous tidal volume $\geq$ 5 mL/kg

3. Minute ventilation $<$ 10 L/min

4. Rapid shallow breathing index $<$ 105

5. Negative inspiratory force $>$ -30 cm H_2O

6. Pao_2 $>$ 58–60 mm Hg

7. pH normal

8. pCO_2 at patient's baseline

---

tracheostomy for prolonged mechanical ventilation will be necessary. In patients with severe disease and/or multiple comorbidities, palliative care should be considered.

PULMONARY REHABILITATION

Pulmonary rehabilitation is an effective and safe intervention for impacting hospital admissions and mortality.[35] Pulmonary rehabilitation is designed to reduce symptoms, optimize function, and improve quality of life. The program should be multidisciplinary and include activity, educational, nutritional, and psychosocial support. Complementary measures to relieve dyspnea and address and improve quality of life and functional capacity should include not only exercise, oxygen, and pharmacotherapeutics but also relaxation techniques, walking aids, sleep aids, and other symptomatic treatments.[36]

Nursing interventions for breathlessness have been tested with mixed effect. The acronym BREATH AIR[36] has been developed to help bedside nurses identify causes and treatments for dyspnea: **B**ronchospasm, **R**ales, **E**ffusions, **A**irway obstruction, **T**hick secretions, **H**emoglobin low, **A**nxiety, **I**nterpersonal issues and **R**eligious concerns have been identified as causes for dyspnea. Appropriate interventions should include pharmacotherapeutics such as steroids and bronchodilators, diuretics, thoracentesis, cough assist devices, mucolytics, suction techniques, transfusions, position, and opioids for physical symptoms. Nursing interventions with emphasis on social, spiritual, and financial support needs to be included in the care planning for effective rehabilitation.[36]

For patients successfully treated and discharged from the ICU, discharge planning should involve a comprehensive evidence-based program. Collaboration with the primary care provider is of utmost importance here. Hopkinson and colleagues[37] developed and piloted a promising care bundle for COPD discharge planning. The program had six components including a referral to a clinical nurse specialist; smoking cessation; rehabilitation referral; demonstration of inhaler use; a follow-up appointment; and information regarding COPD self-management, oxygen therapy, and support groups. The 30-day readmission rate for those receiving the bundle interventions was encouraging with a downward trend, although not statistically significant.[37]

PALLIATIVE AND ADVANCED CARE PLANNING

When NPPV or an attempt at weaning from mechanical ventilation fail or intubation is not an option (for reasons such as patient's wishes, terminal condition), comfort care should be instituted. The progressive nature of the disease and its multisystem effects increase the risk for respiratory failure and death. Patients who refuse life supportive care or request to have it withdrawn require expert delivery of palliative care with interventions, such as dyspnea management and terminal sedation.[1] Discussion of advance directives and advanced care planning (ACP) and referral to the palliative care team assist in decisions regarding supportive care at the end of life (EOL) in patients with COPD admitted to the ICU in acute respiratory failure.

The high burden of the symptoms with COPD, especially dyspnea, reduces overall functional capacity. Discussion of palliative care, symptom relief, quality of life, and improving function should be considered, preferably before requiring ICU admission with ongoing discussion during the ICU admission. Discussion of EOL wishes and advanced directives is imperative as a major element in the comprehensive care of the COPD patient. Curative and restorative care must include palliative care. The American Thoracic Society published an official statement in 2007 that endorses the concepts of palliative care for respiratory disease in critical illness. The statement applies to all stages of COPD and provides recommendations for incorporation of palliative care into treatment, suggested competencies for decision making as well as relationship and communication competencies of health care providers.[38]

ACP, with inclusion of the patient's primary care providers, the patient, and family and/or care givers, is necessary with disease progression of COPD. The aim of ACP should be to increase discussion and increase communication of understanding of the patient's values and goals related to his or her disease. Measures of quality of life and care goals should focus on symptoms including fatigue and dyspnea, activity alterations, emotional function, social isolation, and the patient's perception of the degree of control over the disease.[36]

Heffner[39] discusses the need for ACP and the lack of ACP with COPD patients. Patients with COPD have worse health status, higher functional dependence, and higher levels of anxiety and depression than patients with lung cancer and yet receive less direction and management of EOL care or palliative management.[39] Evaluation of ACP in COPD patients reveals that COPD patients receive insufficient integration of palliative care with disease-directed treatments, which could improve the quality of life.[39] Practitioner reluctance and skill in conducting ACP as well as patient denial, poor understanding of his or her disease, and misperceptions of ACP are barriers to development of EOL care in COPD patients.

Models for implementation of palliative care have suggested that the discussion concerning palliative care occur upon diagnosis or early identification of the disease and well before admission to ICU. Disease-directed treatments with patient-centered goals are identified in these models.[39,40] Multiple diagnostic criteria and clinical prediction instruments have been developed with some promise for tools that will aid practitioners in prognostication. No clear-cut guidelines or measurements have shown consistent outcomes and all need additional testing. Instruments such as the early incorporation of palliative care teams may aid in overcoming barriers to disease management and improved quality of life. Further research is necessary to improve the incorporation of palliative care, identifying triggers in the patient's disease progress that would prompt the practitioner to initiate the discussion.

SUMMARY

Acute exacerbation of COPD resulting in acute respiratory failure is commonly encountered in the ICU. In conjunction with medical therapy, ventilatory support, both noninvasive and invasive, can be lifesaving. However, mechanical ventilation in these patients can be associated with significant adverse consequences, for example, pneumonia, barotrauma, and deconditioning. It is important for caregivers in the ICU to be familiar with the respiratory mechanics in COPD so that appropriate ventilatory settings can be applied for optimal treatment of the respiratory failure. Quality of life and palliative care must be integrated into the care of all COPD patients to address the symptomatic needs of these complex patients.

REFERENCES

1. Global Initiative for Chronic Obstructive Lung Disease (GOLD). Global strategy for the diagnosis, management and prevention of COPD. Available at: http://www.goldcopd.org/. Accessed June 14, 2012.
2. Celli BR, MacNee W, Agusti A, et al. Standards for the diagnosis and management of patients with COPD—a summary of the ATS/ERS position paper. Eur Respir J 2004;23:932–46.
3. Cote C, Celli B. Predictors of mortality in chronic obstructive pulmonary disease. Clin Chest Med 2007;28(3):515.
4. Garvey C. Best practices in chronic obstructive pulmonary disease. Nurse Pract 2011;36(5):16–23.
5. Hanania NA, Marciniuk DD. A unified front against COPD: clinical practice guidelines from the American College of Physicians, the American College of Chest Physicians, the American Thoracic Society, and the European Respiratory Society. Chest 2011; 140(3):565–6.
6. Mannino D, Homa DM, Akinbami LJ, et al. Chronic obstructive pulmonary disease surveillance, United States 1971–2000. MMWR Morb Mortal Wkly Rep 2002;51: 1–16.
7. Shapiro S, Reilly J, Rennard S. Chronic bronchitis and emphysema. In: Mason RJ, Broaddus C, Martin T, et al, editors. Murray and Nadel's textbook of respiratory medicine. 5th edition. Philadelphia: Saunders Elsevier.
8. Rabe KF, Hurd S, Anzueto A, et al. Global strategy for the diagnosis, management, and prevention of chronic obstructive pulmonary disease. Am J Respir Crit Care Med 2007;17:532–55.
9. Celli BR, Cote CG, Marin JM, et al. The body-mass index, airflow obstruction, dyspnea, and exercise capacity index in chronic obstructive pulmonary disease. N Engl J Med 2004;350:1005–12.
10. Emerman CL, Effron D, Lukens TW. Spirometric criteria for hospital admission of patients with acute exacerbations of COPD. Chest 1991;99:595–9.
11. Miravitlles M, Guerrero T, Mayordomo C, et al; EOLO Study Group. Factors associated with increased risk of exacerbation and hospital admission in a cohort of ambulatory COPD patients: a multiple logistics regression analysis. Respiration 2000; 67:495–501.
12. Perera PN, Armstrong EP, Sherrill DL, et al. Acute exacerbations of COPD in the United States: inpatient burden and predictors of costs of mortality. COPD 2012;9: 131–41.
13. Hurst JR, Vestbo J, Anzueto A, et al. Susceptibility to exacerbation in chronic obstructive pulmonary disease. N Engl J Med 2010;363:1128–38.

14. Turner MO, Patel A, Ginsburg S, et al. Bronchodilator delivery in acute airflow Obstruction: a meta-analysis. Arch Intern Med 1997;157:1736–44.
15. Karpel JP, Pesin J, Greenberg D, et al. A comparison of the effects of ipratropium bromide and metaproterenol sulfate in acute exacerbation of COPD. Chest 1990;98: 835–9.
16. Hudson LD, Monti M. Rationale and use of corticosteroids in chronic obstructive pulmonary disease. Med Clin North Am 1990;74:661–90.
17. Davies L, Angus RM, Calverley PM. Oral corticosteroids in patients admitted to hospital with exacerbations of chronic obstructive pulmonary disease: a prospective randomized controlled trial. Lancet 1999;345:456–60.
18. Anthonisen NR, Manfreda J, Warren CPW, et al. Antibiotic therapy in exacerbations of chronic obstructive pulmonary disease. Ann Intern Med 1987;106:196–204.
19. Saint SK, Bent S. Vittinghoff E, et al. Antibiotics in chronic obstructive pulmonary disease exacerbations: a meta-analysis. JAMA 1995;273:957–60.
20. Esper AM, Martin GS. The impact of comorbid conditions on critical illness. Crit Care Med 2011;39(12):2728–35.
21. British Thoracic Society Standards of Care Committee. BTS guideline: noninvasive ventilation in acute respiratory failure. Thorax 2002;57:192–211.
22. Mehta S, Hill NS. Noninvasive ventilation: state of the art. Am J Respir Crit Care Med 2001;163:540–77.
23. International Consensus Conferences in Intensive Care Medicine. Noninvasive positive pressure ventilation in acute respiratory failure. Am J Respir Crit Care Med 2001;163:283–91.
24. Lightowler JV, Wedzicha JA, Elliot M, et al. Noninvasive positive pressure ventilation to treat respiratory failure resulting from exacerbations of chronic obstructive pulmonary disease: Cochrane systematic review and meta-analysis. BMJ 2003;326:185–9.
25. Peter JV, Moran JL, Philips-Hughes J, et al. Noninvasive ventilation in acute respiratory failure: a meta-analysis update. Crit Care Med 2002;30:555–62.
26. Keenan S, Sinuff T, Cook DJ, et al. Which patients with acute exacerbation of chronic obstructive pulmonary disease benefit from noninvasive positive-pressure ventilation? Ann Intern Med 2003;138:861–70.
27. Bott J, Carroll MP, Conway JH, et al. Randomised controlled trial of nasal ventilation in acute ventilatory failure due to chronic obstructive airways disease. Lancet 1993; 341:1555–7.
28. Conti G, Antonelli M, Navalesi P, et al. Noninvaisve vs conventional mechanical ventilation in patients with chronic obstructive pulmonary disease after failure of medical treatment in the ward: a randomized trial. Intensive Care Med 2002;28: 1701–7.
29. Plant PK, Owen JL, Elliott MW. Non-invasive ventilation in acute exacerbations of chronic obstructive pulmonary disease: long term survival and predictors of in-hospital outcome. Thorax 2001;56:708–12.
30. Nava S, Ambrosino N, Clini E, et al. Noninvasive mechanical ventilation in the weaning of patients with respiratory failure due to chronic obstructive pulmonary disease: a randomized study. Ann Intern Med 1998;128:721–8.
31. Ferrer M, Esquinas A, Arancibia F, et al. Noninvasive ventilation during persistent weaning failure. Am J Respir Crit Care Med 2003;168:70–6.
32. Maltais F, Reissmann H, Navalesi P, et al. Comparison of static and dynamic measurements of intrinsic PEEP in mechanically ventilated patients. Am J Respir Crit Care Med 1994;150:1318–24.

33. Reddy RM, Guntupalli KK. Review of ventilatory techniques to optimize mechanical ventilation in acute exacerbation of chronic obstructive pulmonary disease. Int J COPD 2007;2(4):441–52.

34. Puhan MA, Gimeno-Santos E, Scharplatz M, et al. Pulmonary rehabilitation following exacerbations of chronic obstructive pulmonary disease. Cochrane Database Syst Rev 2011;10:CD005305.

35. McCormick JR. Pulmonary rehabilitation and palliative care. Semin Respir Crit Care Med 2009;30(6):684–99.

36. Brennan CW, Mazanec P. Dyspnea management across the palliative care continuum. J Hosp Palliat Nurs 2011;13(3):130–41.

37. Hopkinson NS, Englebretsen C, Cooley N, et al. Designing and implementing a COPD discharge care bundle. Thorax 2012;67(1):90–2.

38. Lanken PN, Terry PB, DeLisser HM, et al. An official American Thoracic Society clinical policy statement: palliative care for patients with respiratory diseases and critical illnesses. Am J Respir Crit Care Med 2008;177:912–27.

39. Heffner JE. Advance care planning in chronic obstructive pulmonary disease: barriers and opportunities. Curr Opin Pulm Med 2011;17(2):103–9.

40. Steer J, Gibson GJ, Bourke SC. Predicting outcomes following hospitalization for acute exacerbations of COPD. QJM 2010;103(11):817–29.

Community-Acquired, Health Care–Associated, and Ventilator-Associated Pneumonia
Three Variations of a Serious Disease

Susan S. Scott, MSN, RN, CCRN[a],*, Cynthia B. Kardos, BSN, RN, BA[b]

KEYWORDS

- Pneumonia • Health care–associated pneumonia • Ventilator-associated pneumonia
- Community-acquired pneumonia • Hospital-acquired pneumonia

KEY POINTS

- Community-acquired pneumonia (CAP), health care–associated pneumonia (HCAP), and ventilator-associated pneumonia (VAP) are three distinct types of pneumonia that cause significant morbidity and mortality.
- Critical care nurses are key members of the health care team in the treatment as well as in the identification and prevention of complications associated with CAP, HCAP, and VAP.

COMMUNITY-ACQUIRED PNEUMONIA

Community-acquired pneumonia (CAP) refers to pneumonia contracted outside the health care setting. According to one estimate noted in the most recent Infectious Disease Society of America/American Thoracic Society (IDSA/ATS) consensus guidelines,[1] 915,900 episodes of CAP occur each year in the United States in adults 65 years of age or older.[2] Furthermore, 20% of all those who develop CAP will require hospitalization, and those with severe CAP may require mechanical ventilation and aggressive multiorgan support.[3]

Clinical Presentation

Clinical presentation of CAP may be typical or atypical. The typical presentation is associated with rapid onset of fever, productive cough, shortness of breath, clinical

The authors have nothing to disclose.
[a] Medical and Surgical Intensive Care Unit, Baystate Medical Center, 759 Chestnut Street, Springfield, MA 01199, USA; [b] Critical Care Research Department, Baystate Medical Center, 759 Chestnut Street, Springfield, MA 01199, USA
* Corresponding author. 63 Pineywoods Avenue, Springfield, MA 01108.
E-mail address: susan.scott@bhs.org

Crit Care Nurs Clin N Am 24 (2012) 431–441
http://dx.doi.org/10.1016/j.ccell.2012.06.003
0899-5885/12/$ – see front matter © 2012 Elsevier Inc. All rights reserved.

signs of pulmonary consolidation (abnormal breath sounds, dullness on percussion), and occasionally pleuritic chest pain.[4] CAP is usually the result of infection by a common bacterial pathogen such as *Streptococcus pneumoniae.* Atypical pneumonia is usually attributed to less common bacterial, viral, and fungal pathogens that colonize in susceptible individuals, such as the elderly or immunocompromised.[5] It has a more gradual onset of dry cough and shortness of breath than typical forms of pneumonia and the patient may experience general myalgias and fatigue.[4] Despite seemingly insignificant pulmonary presentation, the chest radiograph is abnormal in atypical pneumonia.

Causative Organisms

The infecting agent in CAP may be bacterial, viral, or fungal. In otherwise healthy adults (younger than age 60), *Streptococcus pneumoniae* and *Hemophilus influenzae* are common causative agents in CAP.[5] Bacterial agents such as *Mycoplasma pneumoniae, Chlamydia pneumoniae,* and *Legionella pneumophilia* are seen in atypical CAP, as well as viruses (eg, influenza virus, respiratory syncytial virus [RSV], and cytomegalovirus [CMV]). Infections by fungi (eg, *Pneumocystis carinii*) are responsible for a small number of CAP cases and are more likely to occur in immunocompromised patients.[6]

Risk Factors and Severity of CAP

Several different risk factors are associated with CAP, ranging from patient demographics to concomitant illnesses. Currently, the Pneumonia Severity Index (PSI) is one of two main tools available in emergency departments and outpatient settings to determine the severity of CAP. With the PSI model, patient risk scores are determined on the basis of four risk categories: demographic factors, comorbid conditions, findings on physical examination, and laboratory results (eg, pH, blood urea nitrogen [BUN], Sodium, Glucose, hematocrit, and Po_2). Points accumulated within each category are totaled and stratified to one of five risk classes, which correlate to a percent risk of mortality. For a patient with the lowest risk (class I), outpatient treatment is recommended, whereas for a patient found to be at high risk (class IV or V), inpatient treatment is recommended.

The other main pneumonia scoring tool is the CURB65. It is simpler than the PSI and was created for quick and easy use in the emergency department or outpatient office. A patient is assigned 1 point for each of five clinical criteria. A score of 1 or 2 would indicate that an individual can safely be treated as an outpatient, whereas scores of 3 to 5 would suggest inpatient treatment. The five clinical criteria are as follows:

- C   Confusion
- U   Blood urine nitrogen ≥20 mg/dL
- R   Respiratory rate ≥30 breaths/min
- B   Systolic blood pressure <90 mm Hg or diastolic blood pressure ≤60 mm Hg
- 65 Age ≥65 years.

Along with sound clinical judgment, CURB65 and PSI are valuable tools for determining site of care and are strongly recommended by the IDSA)/ATS consensus guidelines.[7] However, recent studies caution that limitations arise when looking at 30-day mortality as an outcome.[8] For example, nearly 50% of pneumonia-related deaths and 25% of deaths occurring within 30 days are related to comorbidities rather than directly caused by pneumonia. These prediction models may underestimate the severity of illness in the young and have been found to perform less well when considering outcomes such as intensive care unit (ICU) admission, mechanical ventilation, and need for vasopressors.[8]

Diagnostic Testing

When a patient is admitted to the hospital for CAP, a chest radiograph should be performed on admission and is essential for detecting pulmonary infiltrates. Complete blood counts and routine chemistries should also be performed, as well as two sets of pretreatment blood cultures. CAP consensus guidelines also support pretreatment Gram stain and culture on expectorated sputum for inpatients. For patients with severe CAP requiring intubation, an endotracheal aspirate for sputum analysis should be obtained.[7] In addition, urinary antigen testing for *Legionella pneumophilia* and *Streptococcus pneumonia* should be performed for patients with severe CAP. If pandemic influenza is suspected, specific flu testing may be indicated.

Treatment and Empiric Therapy

Antibiotic therapy is the main treatment for CAP, with the ultimate goal of killing the infection and resolving the clinical disease. Prompt administration of antibiotic therapy is crucial to favorable CAP outcomes. Early initiation of antibiotics for patients admitted for CAP has been shown to be the single factor most associated with decreased mortality.[9] For patients admitted through the emergency department (ED), the current IDSA/ATS consensus guidelines recommend the first antibiotic dose be administered before the patient leaves the ED.

As a rule, the most potent drugs within a class are preferred, thus helping reduce bacterial selection for antibiotic resistance. Lack of prompt and effective treatment, inappropriate antibiotic choice, or even an insufficient dose with the appropriate antibiotic have all been shown to encourage antibiotic resistance.[3] This may explain why methicillin-resistant *Staphylococcus aureus* (MRSA) has been found to be an occasional causative agent in CAP.

Early in treatment, the infecting agent is often unknown; therefore, broad-spectrum antibiotic therapy may be indicated initially. Empiric antibiotic selection is based on several factors, including age, antibiotic tolerance, comorbidities, concurrent medications, and epidemiologic setting.[5] The IDSA/ATS consensus guidelines make several recommendations based both on patient clinical risks and site of treatment. Intravenous antibiotic therapy is recommended for initial treatment of all individuals requiring inpatient hospital admission, with clear regimen differences between acute and critically ill patients.[7] Once the etiology of CAP has been identified, antimicrobial therapy should be tailored to target the pathogen.

Duration of Treatment

Patients treated with intravenous antibiotics should be switched over to oral medication as soon as clinically possible. This will depend on how the patient is improving clinically, with consideration for such factors as hemodynamic stability, state of the gastrointestinal tract, and ability to ingest medication.[7] According to the IDSA/ATS guidelines, duration of treatment will depend on whether or not the initial antibiotic treatment was active against the infecting pathogen, or if complicating extrapulmonary infections were present. At minimum, 5 days of treatment is recommended; the patient must not only be afebrile for 48 to 72 hours, but must also meet no more than one CAP-associated sign of instability.[7] The following are criteria for clinical instability in CAP:

- Temperature ≥37.8°C
- Heart rate ≥100 beats/min
- Respiratory rate ≥24 breaths/min
- Systolic blood pressure ≤90 mm Hg
- Arterial oxygen saturation ≤90% or P_{O_2} ≤60 mm Hg on room air
- Inability to maintain oral intake
- Normal mental status.

ROLE OF NURSES
Laboratory and Diagnostic Studies

Nurses play a major role in managing the care of CAP patients. They are largely responsible for facilitating the flow of laboratory tests and diagnostic studies in the ward and ICU. Timely collection of specimens and proper techniques for handling of samples are vital to quick and accurate identification of pathogens. This includes practicing good hand hygiene and barrier precautions.

Even though studies have shown that hand hygiene is the single most important method for preventing infection, hand hygiene among health care workers is poor.[10] Compliance has improved somewhat over the last decade, due in large part to the introduction of alcohol-based foams and rubs. However, ongoing surveillance and feedback to nurses and other staff is essential to improving hand hygiene, according to the Centers for Disease Control and Prevention (CDC).[10]

Treatment Failure and Success

In addition to performing frequent physical assessments and overseeing laboratory and diagnostic procedures, nurses must closely monitor a patient's response to treatment. Of CAP patients who die, respiratory failure (along with cardiac arrhythmias and sepsis) is a leading cause of death.[4] A keen ability to recognize new or worsening pulmonary abnormalities, such as hypoxemia, tachypnea, and auscultatory changes, is crucial for identifying treatment failure in CAP.

Recognizing treatment success is important as well, as nurses encourage the patient on the path to recovery. Nurses have the unique privilege of being at the bedside around the clock. They may be the first to recognize when a patient is ready to switch to oral antibiotics, when a central line or indwelling catheter is no longer necessary, or when a patient is ready to leave the ICU. Nurses therefore must be good communicators and facilitators of information to the rest of the clinical team. An important way to do this is to participate in daily rounds.[10]

Patient Education

A key nursing function is to educate patients about their disease throughout the course of treatment and provide them with the necessary information for discharge. Hospital readmissions are common among CAP patients, and most are due to worsening symptoms and comorbidities.[11] Some research has shown that CAP patients have not always been equipped with adequate information for recovery.[12] Patients need to know that their needs are being met and that clinicians are supporting them during their admission. This includes teaching patients the dangerous sign of pneumonia relapse. Patients must be educated on how to recognize fever, worsening cough, and changes in sputum and whom to contact in the event of worsening symptoms. Clinicians may educate best when working within evidence-based guidelines, and when they receive feedback on their performance and that of their peers.[12]

Influenza plays a major part in CAP education. It is estimated that a yearly flu shot can be 70% to 90% effective in preventing influenza.[5] A patient's flu vaccination status should be addressed in the outpatient office and on hospital admission. Education should focus on the preventive health benefits of the flu shot and stress its importance in lowering the risk of influenza pneumonia and secondary bacterial pneumonias, which are more prevalent during flu season.[5] Influenza vaccination should be offered to patients receiving outpatient treatment, as well as at hospital discharge.

Of equal importance is the immunization of health care workers. All clinical personnel in inpatient, outpatient, and long-term care settings should be immunized annually. Influenza vaccination for health care workers is strongly recommended by the current IDSA/ATS consensus guidelines.[7]

HEALTH CARE–ASSOCIATED PNEUMONIA

With the shift of patient care from the hospital into the community, there are many patients receiving extensive health care interventions either in their homes or extended care facilities who may develop pneumonia. This has given rise to a relatively new category of pneumonia termed "health care–associated pneumonia" (HCAP). HCAP is a distinct category of pneumonia. It affects a different patient population than CAP, and the causative organisms differ from those seen with CAP. HCAP is seen in nonhospitalized patients who develop pneumonia and meet one or more of the following criteria: residents in a nursing home or other long-term care facility; receiving invasive treatment (eg, intravenous therapy, hemodialysis, wound care, or intravenous chemotherapy) within 30 days of the onset of the infection; hospitalization in an acute care hospital for two or more days within the prior 90 days; and/or attendance at a hospital within the prior 30 days or a respiratory related problem.

Causative Organisms

Various causative organisms are associated with HCAP owing to the broad cross section of patients in this category. Many patients with recent or chronic contact with the health care system may be at an increased risk for infection by multidrug-resistant organisms.[13] The most common (29%) isolated pneumonia pathogen among those with HCAP in one long-term care facility was *Staphylococcus aureus*, while in those with CAP, *Streptococcus pneumonia* was the predominant (14%) organism.[14] Patients receiving dialysis are often colonized with a multidrug-resistant organism. A review of infections over 9 years in a chronic dialysis unit at a single hospital revealed that the most common causative organisms were *Staphylococcus aureus*, specifically methicillin-resistant *Staphylococcus aureus* (MRSA), *Pseudomonas aeruginosa*, *Klebsiella* species, *Enterobacter* species, and *Escherichia coli*.[15] Influenza A is a common cause of viral HCAP, and immunocompromised patients may develop fungal pneumonias.[13] Therefore, the type of organism may depend not only upon the setting from which the patient has come, but also the local patterns of infection and resistance.

Treatment and Empirical Therapy

As with CAP, antibiotics are key to the treatment of HCAP. The challenge arises in the proper selection of antibiotic therapy for HCAP. The 2005 IDSA/ATS guidelines recommend initiation of empirical antibiotics, although they recognize that this might result in some patients being given antibiotics for a noninfectious process. The benefits of early treatment, however, outweigh this risk. For this reason, de-escalation of antibiotics occurs as soon as clinical assessment indicates resolution of infection and/or cultures dictate a different course of antibiotics.

HOSPITAL-ACQUIRED PNEUMONIA AND VENTILATOR-ASSOCIATED PNEUMONIA

Hospital-acquired pneumonia (HAP, or nosocomial pneumonia) is pneumonia that occurs 48 hours or more after admission to the hospital with no indication of its presence at the time of admission. VAP is a type of HAP that develops more than 48 hours after endotracheal intubation. Because only about 10% of patents with HAP are not mechanically ventilated, the terms HAP and VAP are often used interchangeably.[16]

VAP is the most common nosocomial infection seen in patients in the ICU. Because patients who develop VAP have an increased length of stay by as much as 9 days, an increased cost of care, and possibly mortality rates, compared to critical care patients who do not develop VAP, prevention of this hospital-acquired infection (HAI) is on the forefront of many critical care clinicians' minds.[16] Critical care nurses play a unique role in the prevention of this HAI, as many of the interventions thought to prevent VAP are part of daily nursing care in the ICU.

Diagnosis

According to the CDC guidelines, pneumonia is considered "ventilator associated" if it developed while the patient was intubated and ventilated, or within 48 hours before the onset of the event. There is no minimum amount of time that the ventilator needs to be in place for the pneumonia to be considered ventilator associated. The diagnosis of pneumonia is not a simple one. Diagnosis of VAP can be difficult because several of the clinical indicators are nonspecific, such as fever and elevated or depressed white blood cell count. Purulent sputum is seen not only with pneumonia, but can also be seen with tracheobronchitis. Pulmonary infiltrates are not only present with pneumonia, but can also be associated with atelectasis and acute respiratory distress syndrome.[17]

Types of VAP

VAP is divided into two types: early and late onset. If the occurs pneumonia between 48 and 96 hours after intubation, it is considered an early-onset VAP. Early-onset VAP is usually caused by antibiotic-sensitive organisms. If the VAP develops 96 hours after intubation, it is considered late onset and the causative organisms are usually antibiotic resistant. This later onset VAP is associated with a higher morbidity and mortality rate than the early-onset form.[1]

Incidence

VAP is the most frequently occurring hospital acquired infection. In 2010, the institutions that report to the National Healthcare Safety Network, an infection surveillance program of the CDC, reported more than 3500 cases of VAP in the United States.[18] This infection causes more deaths than central line infections and can add as much as $40,000 to the cost of a hospital stay.[19]

Causes of VAP

The key to the development of VAP is the aspiration of colonized, potentially pathogenic bacteria from the upper respiratory tract and the stomach. Normally, there is clearance of mucus (and the particles and organisms it contains) from the respiratory tract via coughing and mucociliary clearance of secretions. But the presence of the inflated cuff on an endotracheal tube or tracheostomy tube impairs these protective mechanisms. The presence of a nasogastric or orogastric tube disrupts the gastroesophageal sphincter. Secretions from the oropharynx as well as from the stomach (via gastric reflux) collect in the subglottic space above the cuff and are then aspirated. For example, the presence of the cuff protects against macroscopic aspiration, but not against microscopic aspiration.[20,21] The seriousness of this aspiration is compounded by the colonization of pathogenic organisms in the secretions of the mouth and oropharynx, which occurs in patients in ICUs.[22,23]

Another contributing factor in the development of VAP is dental plaque, which can be a reservoir for potential respiratory pathogens. It develops in mechanically ventilated patients because of lack of chewing and in the absence of saliva. Other factors associated with the development of VAP include age greater than 60 years, chronic obstructive pulmonary disease, multiorgan system failure, and head trauma.[24]

Vap Prevention

Because VAP is associated with poor outcomes, including increased length of time on a ventilator, cost of care, morbidity, and mortality, research has been conducted to identify interventions that can prevent its development. In 2005, the Institute of Health Care Improvement (IHI) began its "100,000 Lives" campaign to encourage hospitals and health care providers to reduce harm and deaths. Part of this campaign included the prevention of VAP through the implementation of a group (or bundle) of research-based interventions.[25]

Components of the VAP bundle

There are five key components to the IHI VAP bundle: (1) head of bed elevation, (2) sedation vacation, (3) oral decontamination, (4) peptic ulcer prophylaxis, and (5) deep vein thrombosis prophylaxis. Other interventions include subglottic use of endotracheal tubes that allow for constant or intermittent subglottic suctioning and endotracheal tubes that have an antimicrobial coating. The role of nurses in VAP prevention is discussed, addressing the first three interventions.

Head of bed elevation Because aspiration has been linked to the development of VAP, patient positioning is an important intervention in VAP prevention. It is recommended that the head of the bed (HOB) be elevated because aspiration may be decreased by semirecumbent positioning, particularly in patients receiving enteral feeds. The literature is clear that the supine positioning should be avoided in patients receiving enteral feedings, but it is less clear as to the optimal angle of elevation.[26,27] The IHI VAP bundle cites at least a 30° angle. A study using radioactive labeled enteral feedings found that endotracheal readings were higher in patients who were completely supine compared to those whose head of bed was at 45°. Three studies[28–30] examining positioning all used a maximum HOB elevation of 45°. There is no research, however, describing what the minimal angle of HOB elevation can safely be for the prevention of VAP. Care should be taken with HOB elevation, as there can be skin shearing as a result of the patient sliding down in the bed. This may occur less often if the HOB is at a 30° rather than at a 45° angle. When helping pull the patient up in the bed, utilizing an adequate amount of staff may reduce shearing and will reduce the risk of injury to the ICU staff. Compliance with HOB elevation can be monitored by regular rounding by the charge nurse and educational reinforcement of the importance of elevation. In addition, HOB elevation should be maintained if a patient is transported off of the unit for any reason.

Sedation vacation Because the presence of an endotracheal tube predisposes a patient to VAP, the sooner the patient can be weaned from the ventilator the better.[31]

Oversedation has been shown to increase time on the ventilator and increase ICU stay. Stopping or interrupting the sedation on a daily basis has been shown to reduce these times.[32] The nurse should be present when the sedation is reduced to monitor for ventilator asynchrony and possible oxygen desaturation. Care needs to be taken to monitor the patient during the sedation vacation to avoid the development of agitation and possible self-extubation. It has been shown that those who did not have a sedation vacation had a slightly higher self-extubation rate than those for whom sedation was stopped.[32] In addition, family members visiting during a sedation vacation should be aware of the plan to withdraw sedation and the purpose for doing so. They may be able to provide emotional support to the patient during this period. Once the patient is "lightened up," assessment of readiness to wean can be done. This means that before the sedation vacation coordination with the personnel managing the ventilator at the time needs to occur.

Mouth care In 2010, IHI added the use of chlorhexidine (CHG) for oral decontamination. Mouth care twice daily using a CHG oral rinse was shown to reduce VAP rates in patients who underwent cardiac surgery.[33] Care should be taken to ensure that nurses regularly and correctly. Staff may need to be educated about proper application of the CHG to the oral cavity. Unlike moistening the mouth with water for comfort, the nurse must be sure that the CHG comes in contact with the entire oral cavity. Also, suctioning of excess CHG should be performed to avoid inadvertent aspiration or swallowing of drug.

Other interventions for VAP prevention

Other interventions to prevent VAP include strict hand washing; tooth brushing twice daily to reduce plaque formation on teeth; and suctioning the oropharynx, particularly before repositioning the patient, as often the HOB is lowered to turn and reposition.

NURSING CARE
Physical Assessment

Frequent assessment of breath sounds should be performed to identify any new abnormal sounds as well as to assess improvement of aeration. Clearance of secretions should be facilitated either by encouraging coughing and deep breathing or, if the patient is intubated, performing endotracheal suctioning as needed. Assessment of the character and quality of secretions is also important. Particular attention should be paid to very thick secretions that may result in plugging of the airways. Clinicians should ensure adequate hydration to facilitate clearance of secretions.

Identification of Complications and Treatment Failure

Early identification of treatment failure can help ensure that interventions and therapies are modified in a timely manner to address changes in the patient's condition. Because pneumonia is one of the leading causes of sepsis, vital signs should be monitored with particular attention paid to the early indicators of sepsis (eg, fever, heart rate [HR], etc).[34] Monitoring oxygenation via pulse oximetry should be performed along with the vital signs. Ventilator changes should be made based on changes in oxygenation and ventilation.

Early Ambulation

Promoting progressive ambulation is important as well. Research has shown that patients who ambulate regularly have shorter lengths of stay than those who do not.[4]

Early ambulation while still on the ventilator may also help in the reduction of the neuromuscular complications of critical illness.[35] For those patients unable to ambulate, physical therapy should be instituted, including range-of-motion activities.

Family Participation

Family members wishing to participate in care may be educated in proper performance range-of-motion activities, rotation of splints, and mouth care. Participation in care allows family members to feel as though they are supporting the recovery of their loved one. This is particularly true if family members have been caretakers of the patient before admission to the hospital.

Patient and Family Education

Another key nursing function is patient and family education. Individuals 50 years or older, those at high risk for influenza complications, and those who have household contact with high-risk individuals should be encouraged to obtain an annual influenza vaccine. The pneumococcal vaccine should be recommended for individuals 65 years of age or older and those with concomitant high risk diseases.[7] Patient education must include support around smoking cessation strategies so they may be successful in quitting.

SUMMARY

CAP, HCAP, and VAP are three distinct types of pneumonia that cause significant morbidity and mortality. Critical care nurses are key members of the health care team in the treatment as well as in the identification and prevention of complications associated with CAP, HCAP, and VAP.

REFERENCES

1. American Thoracic Society, Infectious Diseases Society of America. Guidelines for the management of adults with hospital acquired, ventilator associated and healthcare associated pneumonia. Am J Respir Crit Care Med 2005;171:388–416.
2. Jackson ML, Neuzil KM, Thompson WW, et al. The burden of community-acquired pneumonia in seniors: results of a population based study. Clin Infec Dis 2004; 39:1642–50.
3. Shah PB, Meleveedu R, Elayaraja S, et al. Interventions for treating community-acquired pneumonia: an overview of the cochrane systematic reviews (protocol). Cochrane Database Syst Rev 2011;10.
4. Kleinpell RM, Elpern EH. Community-acquired pneumonia: updates in assessment and management. Crit Care Nur Q 2004;27:231–40.
5. Boldt MD, Kiresuk T. Community-acquired pneumonia in adults. Nurs Pract 2001;26: 14–23.
6. Shultz TR. On the trail of community-acquired pneumonia. Nurs Manage 2003;34(2 Pt 1):27–32.
7. Mandell LA, Wunderink RG, Anzueto A, et al. Infectious Disease Society of America/ American Thoracic Society consensus guidelines on the management of community-acquired pneumonia in adults. Clin Infect Dis 2007;44(Suppl 2):S27–72.
8. Chalmers JD. ICU admission and severity assessment in community-acquired pneumonia. Crit Care 2009;13(3):156.
9. Meehan TP, Fine MJ, Krumholz HM, et al. Quality of care, process and outcomes in elderly patients with pneumonia. JAMA 1997;278:2080–4.

10. Aragon D, Sole ML. Implementing best practice strategies to prevent infection in the ICU. Crit Care Nurs Clin North Am 2006;18:441–52.
11. Adamuz J, Viasus D, Camprecios-Rodriguez P, et al. A prospective cohort study of healthcare visits and rehospitalizations after discharge of patients with community-acquired pneumonia. Respirology 2011;16(7):1119–26.
12. Horowitz CR, Chassin MR. Improving the quality of pneumonia care that patients experience. Am J Med 2002;113:379–83.
13. Falcone M, Vendetti M, Yuichiro S. et al. Healthcare associated pneumonia: diagnostic criteria and distinction from community acquired pneumonia. Int J Infect Dis 2011;15(8):e545–50.
14. El Solh AA, Pietrantoni C, Bhat A et al. Indicators of potentially drug resistant bacteria in severe nursing home acquired pneumonia. Clin Infect Dis 2004;39:474–80.
15. Berman SJ, Johnson EW, Nakatsu C, et al. Burdens of infection in patients with end stage renal disease requiring long term dialysis. Clin Infect Dis 2004;39:1747–53.
16. Wood GC, Swanson JM. Managing ventilator-associated pneumonia. AACN Adv Crit Care 2009;20(4):309–16.
17. Institute for Healthcare Improvement. How-to guide: prevent ventilator-associated pneumonia. Available at: http://www.ihi.org. Accessed March 24, 2012.
18. Dudeck MA, Horan TC, et al. National Healthcare Safety Network (NHSN) report: data summary for 2010. Available at: http://www.cdc.gov/nhsn/PDFs/dataStat/2011NHSNReport.pdf. Accessed March 20, 2012.
19. Zilberberg MD, Shorr AF. Ventilator associated pneumonia a model for approaching cost-effectiveness and infection prevention in the ICU. Curr Opin Infect Dis 2011;24(4):385–9.
20. Berra L, Sampson J, Fumagalli J, et al. Alternative approach to ventilator associated pneumonia prevention. Minerva Anestesiol 2011;77:323–33.
21. Muscedere J, Rewa O, Mckechnie K, et al. Subglottic secretion drainage for the prevention of ventilator-associated pneumonia: a systematic review and meta-analysis Crit Care Med 2011;39(8):1985–91.
22. Kallet RH, Quinn THE. The gastrointestinal tract and ventilator associated pneumonia. Respir Care 2005;50:910–21.
23. Torres A, Serra-Batlles J, Ros E, et al. Pulmonary aspiration of gastric contents in patient receiving mechanical ventilation: the effect of body position. Ann Intern Med 1992;116 540–3.
24. Bonten MJ, Kollef MH, Hall JB. Risk factors for ventilator associated pneumonia: from epidemiology to patient management. Clin Infect Dis 2004;38(8):1141–9.
25. Lawrence P, Fulbrook P. The ventilator care bundle and its impact on ventilator associated pneumonia: a review of the evidence. Nurs Crit Care 2011;16(5):222–34.
26. Bonten M. Healthcare epidemiology: ventilator associated pneumonia: preventing the inevitable. Clin Infect Dis 2011;52:115–21.
27. Bassi GL, Torres A. Ventilator associated pneumonia: role of positioning. Curr Opin Crit Care 2011;17:57–63.
28. Drakulovic MB, Torres A, Bauer TT, et al. Supine body position as a risk factor for nosocomial pneumonia in mechanically ventilated patients: a randomized trial. Lancet 1999;354:1851–8.
29. Van Nieuwenhoven CA, Vandenbroucke-Grauls C, van Tiel FH, et al. Feasibility and effects of the semirecumbent position to prevent ventilator associated pneumonia: a randomized control study. Crit Care Med 2006;34:396–402.
30. Keely L. Reducing the risk of ventilator acquired pneumonia through head of bed elevation. Nurs Crit Care 2007;12:287–94.

31. Koenig SM, Truwit JD. Ventilator-associated pneumonia: diagnosis, treatment, and prevention. Clin Microbiol 2006;19(4):637–57.
32. Kress JP, Pohlman AS, O'Connor MF, et al. Daily interruption of sedative infusions in critically ill patients undergoing mechanical ventilation. N Engl J Med 2000;342: 1471–7.
33. DeRiso AJ 2, Ladowski JS, Dillon TA, et al. Chlorhexidine gluconate 0.12% oral rinse reduces the incidence of total nosocomial respiratory infection and nonprophylactic systemic antibiotic use in patients undergoing heart surgery. Chest 1996;109(6): 1556–61.
34. Kellum JA, Kong L. Understanding the inflammatory cytokine response in pneumonia and sepsis. Arch Intern Med 2007;167(15):1655–63.
35. Bailey, P Thomsen, GE. Early activity is feasible and safe in respiratory failure patients. Crit Care Med 2007;35(1):139–45.

Understanding Advanced Modes of Mechanical Ventilation

Shannon Johnson Bortolotto, RN, MS, CCNS[a],*,
Mary Beth Flynn Makic, RN, PhD, CNS, CCNS, CCRN[a,b]

KEYWORDS

- Mechanical ventilation • Pressure ventilation • Noninvasive ventilation
- Lung protective strategy • Open lung • Alveolar recruitment maneuvers

KEY POINTS

- Approaches to mechanical ventilation (MV) are consistently changing, and the level of ventilator sophistication provides opportunities to improve pulmonary support for critically ill patients.
- Advanced MV modes are used in the treatment of patients with complex pulmonary conditions.
- This article describes the evidence supporting advanced lung protective modes of MV used in the care of critically ill adults.

INTRODUCTION

Critical care nurses should understand the concepts of mechanical ventilation (MV), as an effective management strategy for patients requiring MV that can influence morbidity and mortality in the ICU environment. A classic study by Gajic and colleagues[1] demonstrated that injudicious MV resulted in damage to the pulmonary tissue in as little as 30 minutes. This tissue injury created an alveolar inflammatory response resulting in poor lung function.[1] Integrating evidence-based knowledge and skill related to MV is necessary to maximize the benefits of this intervention in the support of critically ill patients.

Approaches to optimal MV management are constantly being evaluated and refined. In the past decade, ventilators have become more sophisticated, and now can respond to patient-initiated breaths while modifying both pressure and volume in response to changing pulmonary dynamics. This allows for advanced MV modes to be utilized in the treatment of patients with complex pulmonary conditions.[2] Paired

The authors have nothing to disclose.
[a] Critical Care, University of Colorado Hospital, 12605 East 16th Avenue Aurora, CO 80045, USA;
[b] University of Colorado, College of Nursing, Anschutz Medical Campus, Aurora, CO 80045, USA
* Corresponding author. 4200 Julian Street, Denver, CO 80211.
E-mail address: shannon.johnson@uch.edu

with MV sophistication is a need for critical care nurses to integrate pulmonary and MV knowledge in the care of critically ill patients. The purpose of this article is to discuss the principles of MV, clinical indications, and the relevant evidence-based literature supporting lung protective strategies of MV in the care of critically ill adults. The assumption is that the reader has a working knowledge of basic MV principles (eg, pressure support [PS], continuous positive airway pressure [CPAP], assist control [AC], controlled mechanical ventilation [CMV], synchronized intermittent mandatory ventilation [SIMV], and intermittent mandatory ventilation [IMV]).

PRINCIPLES AND EFFECTS OF MV

Effective management of patients requiring MV depends on the clinician's knowledge of normal pulmonary physiology and mechanics of breathing. The pulmonary system is a low-pressure system that serves two essential physiologic functions: oxygenation and ventilation. Both of these processes require effective pulmonary function paired with adequate perfusion of the lungs. Breathing naturally, without the assistance of MV, is achieved by negative inspiratory force mechanics. During inspiration the diaphragm and accessory muscles contract, generating a negative pressure, pulling air in. Relaxation of the diaphragm and other muscles allows air to passively leave the lungs. An intact circulation surrounding the alveoli, matched to functional alveoli, results in optimal diffusion of oxygen (O_2) and carbon dioxide (CO_2).

Inspiratory assistance with MV completely "flips" the natural mechanics of negative pressure inspiration. MV breaths are delivered by positive pressure, thereby "pushing" air into the lungs. Pulmonary surfactant is a mixture of lipids and proteins that line the alveolus lowering surface tension and maintains alveolar surface area for effective gas exchange in the healthy lung.[3] Pulmonary disease, inflammatory triggers, and the positive pressure mechanics of MV disrupt the balance of surfactant necessary to maintain open alveoli.[4] Disruption in the surfactant–alveoli interface causes atelectasis that results in a ventilation/perfusion mismatch. A pulmonary shunt is described as a diffusion or perfusion impairment resulting in decreased oxygenated blood returning into arterial circulation.[5]

To maximize oxygenation and ventilation for the patient requiring MV, open lung strategies are implemented. Lachmann first described open lung protective therapies in 1992.[6] Open lung strategy refers to employing modes of ventilation that minimize alveolar loss through positive pressure and include the recruitment of collapsed alveoli.[7] This is typically achieved in MV by (1) adjusting the positive end-expiratory pressure (PEEP) to avoid alveolar collapse, (2) using a low peak inspiratory pressure (PIP) to deliver effective breaths, and (3) employing decelerating air flow patterns.[4,7,8] Decelerating air flow patterns refer to the speed of the gas delivered during inspiration and the slow release of the gas, distributing air more effectively as the chest fills before expiration[9] (**Fig. 1**). This flow pattern is considered more physiologic in nature, contributing to better alveoli gas distribution.[4,7–9] Advanced MV modes that incorporate open lung strategies deliver decelerating air flow breaths predominantly using pressure-regulated modes rather than volume (ie, size of tidal volume). Newer and more sophisticated pressure modes of MV have been found to be more effective in maintaining an open lung for maximal alveolar function.[4,9]

The lung is a low-pressure system. By changing the mechanics of breathing during MV to positive pressure, intrathoracic pressures are increased; that is, more force is exerted within the thoracic space than normal. This increased intrathoracic pressure can result in symptoms of hemodynamic instability, notably reduction in cardiac output. Pushing air into the pulmonary system via MV also causes mechanical trauma to the lung, known as *barotrauma*. In fact, the greater the application of pressure to

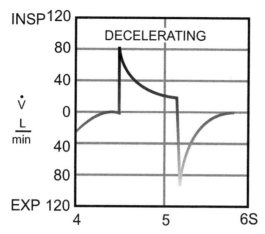

Fig. 1. Decelerating flow waveform. *Abbreviations:* EXP, expiration; INSP, inspiration; S, seconds; V̇, flow. (Image used by permission from Nellcor Puritan Bennett LLC, Boulder, Colorado, doing business as Covidien.)

deliver a breath, the worse the barotrauma (ie, lung damage).[8,10,11] *Volutrauma*, on the other hand, refers to lung damage caused by high tidal volumes. A combination of high tidal volumes and high pressures increases the stress on the pulmonary system and compound tissue injury and barotrauma.[8] This tissue insult activates proinflammatory cytokines, triggering an intrapulmonary inflammatory cascade, referred to as *biotrauma*.[8,12] Cyclic opening and closing of alveoli caused by ineffective MV exacerbates biotrauma and *ventilator induced lung injury* (VILI).[8]

Management of patients on MV attempts to provide effective oxygenation and ventilation with the least amount of pulmonary trauma. This can be accomplished through various advanced modes and settings utilized in mechanical ventilation. MV modes that employ lower tidal volumes, decelerating pressure regulated breaths, and effective PEEP are necessary to minimize VILI and are considered lung protective strategies.[4,8–10]

INDICATIONS FOR MV

Management of patients on MV requires that the critical care nurse appreciate the treatment goals for the intervention as well as the underlying pulmonary disorder(s) (ie, disease/systemic pathology, oxygenation, ventilation or mixed pulmonary disorder). Disturbances in O_2 and CO_2 exchange include both oxygenation and ventilation impairments: apnea, acute or impending ventilatory failure, severe hypoxemia, and respiratory muscle fatigue.[13]

Diffusion concentration gradients perpetuate the movement of both O_2 and CO_2 across the alveolar–capillary membrane. Factors interfering with effective diffusion can originate from disruption of the alveoli, the capillaries surrounding the alveoli, or the insterstitium. Pulmonary edema, inflammation, vasoconstriction, poor ventilation, and poor oxygenation are disruptive to adequate gas diffusion. When factors interfere with effective diffusion through poor ventilation, poor perfusion, or a combination of these factors, deoxygenated hemoglobin returns to the circulatory system, resulting in a physiologic shunt. The most common causes of shunt occur in acute respiratory distress syndrome (ARDS), atelectasis, pneumonia, pulmonary edema, pulmonary embolus, and intracardiac right-to-left flow shunts.

The presence of a shunt is further appreciated when critical care clinicians calculate alveolar–arterial (A–a) gradients, shunted blood flow-to-total blood flow ratio (Q_s/Q_t), arterial to alveolar ratio (Pao_2/PAo_2), or ratio of Pao_2 to fraction of inspired oxygen (F_IO_2) (P/F).[14] Normal physiologic shunt equates to 2% to 5% of the cardiac output via the cardiac venous circulation. Shunting can be estimated noninvasively by examining P/F relationship. Clinical concerns are present when P/F are 300 mm Hg or lower. Oxygen Index (OI) calculation also incorporates the measurement of the severity of oxygenation impairment in combination with the mean airway pressure (mP_{aw}). OI has been classically utilized in the pediatric population, but is gaining momentum in the adult population as a predictor of respiratory outcome. An OI of 20 or greater is associated with increased mortality. A P/F of 100 mm Hg or less and an OI of 30 or greater are considered measures of severe pulmonary dysfunction and a failure of conventional ventilation, which may necessitate lung protective MV modes of ventilation.[15] It is clinically important to conceptualize the underlying cause and complexity of a pulmonary shunt to identify which lung protective mode of MV may be most beneficial to the patient.

MV STRATEGIES

Traditionally, MV included principles of delivering breaths based on volume (eg, size of breath) or pressure. Volume modes would trigger inspiration and the cycling of breaths was based on programmed tidal volume, rate, and time that were believed to provide optimal ventilation. Classic strategies of ventilation (eg, CMV, AC, SIMV, IMV) were programmed irrespective of pulmonary compliance. Although these classic volume modes continue to be used in the short-term management of patients requiring MV support, they have been less effective in providing open lung protective ventilation in critically ill patients.[9] Newer modes of MV based on pressure principles rather than volume provide lower tidal volumes, decelerating air flow patterns, and pressure and maintain open lung ventilation.

Historically higher tidal volume breaths, defined as 10 to 15 mL/kg, were calculated from either actual or predicted body weight to determine the tidal volume setting. Advances in clinical research have demonstrated adverse effects from high tidal volumes shifting this practice. Current practice accepts usage of lower tidal volumes defined as 4 to 8 mL/kg.

A large multicenter research study known as the Acute Respiratory Distress Syndrome Network study (ARDS Net) examined tidal volume (low vs high) in the treatment of patients with ARDS.[15,16] This study defined low tidal volume as 4 to 8 mL/kg and high tidal volume as 12 mL/kg. Patients with ARDS and acute lung injury (ALI) were randomized to receive either high (control group) or low (treatment group) tidal volumes. The study was stopped after the enrollment of 861 patients because of decreased mortality and decreased ventilator days noted in the treatment group (ie, patients receiving low tidal volumes). Findings from this study described that lower tidal volumes protect the lungs from excessive stretch, improving patient outcomes.[16]

A process of incorporating lung protective strategies into clinical practice supports the use of ideal body weight (IBW) as opposed to actual or daily body weight. Tidal volume calculations based on IBW usage at 4 to 8 mL/kg, maintaining plateau pressures at 30 cm of H_2O or lower and incorporating moderate levels of PEEP (ie, 5–15 cm of H_2O).[17] However, if alveolar derecruitment persists, as evidenced by episodes of refractory hypoxemia, careful consideration should be exercised in adjusting to higher levels of PEEP (ie, 15–24 cm H_2O).[14] Excessive alveolar stretch has been shown to cause barotrauma and further compromise atelectatac regions of the lung. The use of lung protective strategies in critical care has been shown to offer a survival benefit, a decrease in ventilatory days, and is currently considered the standard of care[15] (**Fig. 2**).

Beyond the ARDS Net study, there was a recent randomized controlled trial comparing lower tidal volume usage (4–8 mL/kg) versus historically larger tidal volumes (10–15 mL/kg) in patients who do not meet the clinical criteria for ALI. The trial was stopped prematurely because of increased rates of ALI in the higher tidal volume group.[18] These findings support the usage of lower tidal volumes at 4 to 8 mL/kg, calculated from IBW for all mechanically ventilated patients.

Pressure Control Ventilation

Pressure control ventilation (PCV) is increasingly utilized in patients experiencing respiratory failure due to the ability to regulate peak inspiratory pressure, resulting in less barotrauma. Inspiratory air flow patterns are delivered in a decelerated manner in which the pressure necessary to deliver this air is decreased, resulting in a more rapid alveolar fill and equitable gas distribution. Alveoli that were previously collapsed or atelectatac are re-recruited by maintaining an increased pressure throughout the inspiratory cycle. This ventilation mode uses a predetermined inspiratory pressure that is maintained for a set period of time during inspiration. The volume of gas delivered will vary dependent on lung compliance as the tidal volume is determined by the air flow delivered according to the set pressure. For example, if the inspiratory pressure is set at 35 cm H_2O to achieve a tidal volume of 400 mL, as the lungs become less compliant, the MV will continue to deliver gas at 35 cm H_2O, but the tidal volume will decrease. This PCV feature reduces barotrauma but may compromise the size of tidal volume delivered. In addition to setting pressure flow parameters, inspiration and expiration time ratio (I/E ratio) can be adjusted to allow for shortened or longer phases of either of these cycles. Early ventilator modes were not sensitive to spontaneous breaths and therefore delivered pressure on inspiration, irrespective of whether the patient was initiating his own breath. Sedation or neuromuscular blockade pharmacologic agents were often administered to patients for mode tolerance. Current ventilators are more sensitive to spontaneous breathing efforts. Ventilators now sense a patient's spontaneous breath and adjust the gas flow delivered to meet the patient's ventilatory needs.[9]

The goal of PCV is to control airway pressure while meeting ventilation needs. If lung compliance decreases with worsening pulmonary disease, a decrease in tidal volume will occur. Subsequent adjustments in pressure are needed to meet the ventilatory needs of the patient while minimizing barotrauma. The most significant difference between PCV and traditional volume control modes is volume based modes deliver a set tidal volume regardless of pressure required.[19] When PCV is utilized, improved gas exchange occurs, work of breathing decreases and overdistension of alveoli is reduced.[20]

PCV has historically been used in the management of patients with pulmonary diseases that result in poor compliance or "stiff lungs," such as ALI, ARDS, and inhalation injury.[21] Nursing considerations focus on monitoring changes in tidal volume relative to set pressure to meet ventilation and oxygenation goals. Documenting and trending tidal volumes and pressure limits, along with clinical variables such as pulse oximetry trends and arterial blood gas results are required. Initially, cardiac output may fluctuate due to changes in intrathoracic pressure. Thus, trends in blood pressure are important to monitor with increases in pressure in PCV. Because PCV mode may not synchronize with a patient's spontaneous breathing efforts, sedation may be required.

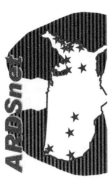

NIH NHLBI ARDS Clinical Network
Mechanical Ventilation Protocol Summary

INCLUSION CRITERIA: Acute onset of

1. $PaO_2/FiO_2 \leq 300$ (corrected for altitude)
2. Bilateral (patchy, diffuse, or homogeneous) infiltrates consistent with pulmonary edema
3. No clinical evidence of left atrial hypertension

PART I: VENTILATOR SETUP AND ADJUSTMENT

1. Calculate predicted body weight (PBW)
   Males = 50 + 2.3 [height (inches) - 60]
   Females = 45.5 + 2.3 [height (inches) -60]
2. Select any ventilator mode
3. Set ventilator settings to achieve initial V_T = 8 ml/kg PBW
4. Reduce V_T by 1 ml/kg at intervals $\leq$ 2 hours until V_T = 6ml/kg PBW.
5. Set initial rate to approximate baseline minute ventilation (not > 35 bpm).
6. Adjust V_T and RR to achieve pH and plateau pressure goals below.

OXYGENATION GOAL: PaO_2 55-80 mmHg or SpO_2 88-95%

Use a minimum PEEP of 5 cm H_2O. Consider use of incremental FiO_2/PEEP combinations such as shown below (not required) to achieve goal.

Lower PEEP/higher FiO2

FiO₂	0.3	0.4	0.4	0.5	0.5	0.6	0.7	0.7
PEEP	5	5	8	8	10	10	10	12

FiO₂	0.7	0.8	0.9	0.9	1.0
PEEP	14	14	14	16	18	18-24

Higher PEEP/lower FiO2

FiO₂	0.3	0.3	0.3	0.3	0.3	0.4	0.4	0.5
PEEP	5	8	10	12	14	14	16	16

FiO₂	0.5	0.5-0.8	0.8	0.9	1.0	1.0
PEEP	18	20	22	22	22	24

PLATEAU PRESSURE GOAL: $\leq$ 30 cm H_2O

Check Pplat (0.5 second inspiratory pause), at least q 4h and after each change in PEEP or V_T.

If Pplat > 30 cm H_2O: decrease V_T by 1ml/kg steps (minimum = 4 ml/kg).

If Pplat < 25 cm H_2O and V_T< 6 ml/kg, increase V_T by 1 ml/kg until Pplat > 25 cm H_2O or V_T = 6 ml/kg.

If Pplat < 30 and breath stacking or dys-synchrony occurs: may increase V_T in 1ml/kg increments to 7 or 8 ml/kg if Pplat remains $\leq$ 30 cm H_2O.

Fig. 2. NIH NHLBI ARDS Clinical Network, mechanical ventilation protocol summary. Available at: http://www.ardsnet.org/system/files/Ventilator%20Protocol%20Card.pdf.

pH GOAL: 7.30-7.45
Acidosis Management: (pH < 7.30)
If pH 7.15-7.30: Increase RR until pH > 7.30 or $PaCO_2 < 25$ (Maximum set RR = 35).

If pH < 7.15: Increase RR to 35.
If pH remains < 7.15, V_T may be increased in 1 ml/kg steps until pH > 7.15 (Pplat target of 30 may be exceeded).
May give $NaHCO_3$
Alkalosis Management: (pH > 7.45) Decrease vent rate if possible.

I: E RATIO GOAL: Recommend that duration of inspiration be ≤ duration of expiration.

PART II: WEANING
A. Conduct a SPONTANEOUS BREATHING TRIAL daily when:
1. $FiO_2 ≤ 0.40$ and PEEP ≤ 8.
2. PEEP and FiO_2 ≤ values of previous day.
3. Patient has acceptable spontaneous breathing efforts. (May decrease vent rate by 50% for 5 minutes to detect effort.)
4. Systolic BP ≥ 90 mmHg without vasopressor support.
5. No neuromuscular blocking agents or blockade.

B. SPONTANEOUS BREATHING TRIAL (SBT):
If all above criteria are met and subject has been in the study for at least 12 hours, initiate a trial of UP TO 120 minutes of spontaneous breathing with FiO2 ≤ 0.5 and PEEP ≤ 5:
1. Place on T-piece, trach collar, or CPAP ≤ 5 cm H_2O with PS ≤ 5
2. Assess for tolerance as below for up to two hours.
   a. $SpO_2 ≥ 90$: and/or $PaO_2 ≥ 60$ mmHg
   b. Spontaneous $V_T ≥ 4$ ml/kg PBW
   c. RR ≤ 35/min
   d. pH ≥ 7.3
   e. No respiratory distress (distress= 2 or more)
   ➤ HR > 120% of baseline
   ➤ Marked accessory muscle use
   ➤ Abdominal paradox
   ➤ Diaphoresis
   ➤ Marked dyspnea
3. If tolerated for at least 30 minutes, consider extubation.
4. If not tolerated resume pre-weaning settings.

Definition of UNASSISTED BREATHING
(Different from the spontaneous breathing criteria as PS is not allowed)

1. Extubated with face mask, nasal prong oxygen, or room air, OR
2. T-tube breathing, OR
3. Tracheostomy mask breathing, OR
4. **CPAP less than or equal to 5 cm H_20 without pressure support or IMV assistance.**

Fig. 2. (continued)

Pressure-Regulated Volume Control

Pressure-regulated volume control (PRVC) combines features of volume control ventilation (set tidal volume) with variable pressures to achieve the desired level of gas exchange.[4,22] With PRVC the ventilator senses inspiratory pressure with each breath. Pressures are increased or decreased, depending on changes in pulmonary compliance and lung mechanics to attain the goal tidal volume. Alarms are triggered if the tidal volume or pressure limits are violated. The ventilator measures the tidal volume on a breath to breath basis, delivering the necessary pressure (within set limits) to achieve the desired tidal volume. In this mode, the nurse should monitor changes in pressure delivered by the ventilator to ensure pressure limit adherence and tidal volume achievement. The nurse should evaluate high pressure alarms and explore decreasing lung compliance, obstructions, or ventilator malfunction. Similar to PCV, this mode may be used in the management of patients with poor lung compliance seen in ALI and ARDS.

Pressure Support Ventilation

Pressure support ventilation (PSV) is used to augment spontaneous breaths initiated by the patient.[22] In this mode, a pressure level is selected that augments or supports spontaneous patient-triggered breaths.[9] When the patient initiates a breath the preset pressure rises quickly, assisting the patient's spontaneous efforts, thereby reducing the work of breathing. The higher the set pressure, the less laborious it is for the patient to initiate a breath[9]; however, as mentioned earlier, high pressures (as well as high volumes) can produce barotrauma. Therefore the threshold for setting pressures, takes into consideration the risk to the patient versus the pressures needed to adequately ventilate the patient.

Because PSV is used for spontaneous breaths, no rate or tidal volume is set. The patient's effort determines the rate of breathing and tidal volume. Pressure settings range from 5 to 20 cm H_2O. PSV can be used as the primary mode of ventilation when weaning. It can also be used in conjunction with volume modes, such as IMV, to support spontaneous breaths between IMV breaths. Nursing care considerations focus on awareness of the PSV pressure set, patient initiated rate, and size of tidal volume. The nurse should monitor for changes in tidal volume as a measure of patient inspiratory effort. As noted with PRVC, the nurse must be able to monitor these changes to ensure adequate ventilation and the significance of alarms. Assessment of breathing effort and fatigue (ie, decreasing tidal volumes, use of accessory muscles such as retraction, neck muscle use, paradoxical respiration, and changes in level of consciousness) are important monitoring principles in the care of a patient using PSV.

Proportional Assist Ventilation

This mode of MV is applied to spontaneously breathing patients and is designed to deliver support based on continuous measurements of the patient's ventilatory support needs.[9] Proportional assist ventilation (PAV) does not set target pressure, volume, or flow rates. Alternately, the ventilator measures throughout the inspiratory/expiratory cycle and automatically adjusts the necessary pressure, airflow, and volume needed to compensate for increased breathing resistance.[9,23] PAV is considered a more physiologic breathing pattern because this mode responds rapidly to changes in ventilation efforts. One study reported increased patient comfort and sleeping patterns in patients on PAV compared to other modes of MV.[24] More studies are needed to determine the use of PAV as a weaning mode as well as in the support of more acutely ill spontaneously breathing patients that require some sort of MV support. [9]

RESCUE MODES OF MV

The term "rescue" modes for MV is used to describe lung protective modes of ventilation that are employed for persistent hypoxemia. Often these patients are suffering from pulmonary derangements including severe refractory hypoxemia as measured by diminished P/F ratios of 100 mm Hg or lower. Rescue modes of ventilation are categorized as airway pressure release ventilation (APRV) and high-frequency oscillatory ventilation (HFOV).[14] A superior rescue mode of ventilation has not yet been established. Clinical usage is influenced by clinician expertise, staff competency, and equipment availability.

Airway Pressure Release Ventilation

Airway pressure release ventilation (APRV), also known as BiPhasic/BiLevel ventilation, is an advanced mode that combines PC with CPAP to support a patient's spontaneous breathing efforts.[9,19,23] For patients experiencing ALI and ARDS, there is an increased effort in work of breathing, a diminished pulmonary compliance and a decreased functional capacity. The use of continuous positive airway pressure (CPAP) in APRV supports spontaneous breathing efforts that result in the employment of dependent alveoli and aids in re-recruitment.[19] So although the patient initiates the breath, the ventilator is continuously delivering some level of pressure within the airways for both inspiration and expiration. This mode incorporates a pressure release phase by applying an active expiratory release option in a pressure low (P_{low}) phase during ventilation. APRV is pressure limited and time cycled based on desired respiratory frequency (eg, set respiratory rate). A short, 1.5- to 2.0-second airway pressure decrease during the P_{low} phase, allows for lung recoil and gas compression energy to aid in increased removal of CO_2.[19] This brief release of pressure is the hallmark of this mode and aids in reducing ventilator dyssynchrony. Ventilation occurs at cycled times that have two variant pressure settings and time settings: CPAP or pressure high (P_{high}) and release phase, or an interruption in CPAP during pressure low (P_{low}). This is combined with time high (T_{high}) and time low (T_{low}) spent at each pressure point. The ventilator-determined tidal volume varies based on lung compliance, airway resistance pressures, and the duration/timing of the pressure release maneuver.[19] When opening pressure is maintained by an increased time, T_{high}, partially collapsed alveoli are enlisted. If alveolar opening pressure is uncertain, this is a chosen mode to assist with CPAP support for spontaneous respirations to maintain consistent alveolar recruitment. The short airway pressure release also permits partial emptying of lung volume, retaining open alveoli. If the patient is not spontaneously breathing, APRV resembles the PC mode of MV.

In contrast to conventional MV, APRV does not raise airway pressures, increase lung volumes, and overdistend the pulmonary infrastructure—all of which result in a potential for increased intrathoracic pressure with diminished cardiac output and hemodynamic instability.[23] APRV potentially decreases some discomfort of ventilation by supporting spontaneous breathing and therefore lessens the problems associated with ventilator dyssynchrony (ie, anxiety with ventilation, over-breathing with less effective support).[19,23] Clinical and experimental studies involving APRV are connected to pulmonary improvement in the management of patients with ALI and ARDS. Common physiologic parameters measured in these failure states include diminished diffusion of gases, ventilation impairments, and cardiac output deficiencies, all of which have been shown to be improved end point markers with APRV.[19] Further studies are needed that compare the usage of APRV with oxygenation improvements as well as reduce mortality, ICU length of stay, and days to ventilator liberation.[25]

Nursing considerations for the care of patients on APRV require knowledge of the set frequency of ventilation, CPAP supported spontaneous efforts by the patient, tidal volumes (mechanical and spontaneous breaths), and mean airway pressures that reflect changes in lung compliance. Ideally in PRVC, synchrony with the ventilator is enhanced along with improved gas exchange (ie, improved oxygenation and CO_2 removal).

High-Frequency Oscillatory Ventilation

High-frequency oscillatory ventilation (HFOV) in adults is increasingly used as a lung protective strategy in critically ill patients.[25,26] It is a mode that has been clinically studied, is safe to use in clinical practice, and has a potential for improved survivability in ALI and ARDS if used early.[27]

HFOV is defined as a mode of MV that delivers a high-amplitude tidal volume, ranging from 1 to 3 mL/kg[25] to minimize alveolar overdistension, in combination with the maintenance of a high end-expiratory lung pressure to decrease alveolar collapse.[28] High rates (300–420 breaths/min [bpm]), coupled with high-frequency (3–7 Hertz [Hz]) oscillations, create pressure waves that enhance CO_2 elimination and improve oxygenation via the establishment of a constant mP_{aw}. One Hz is equal to 60 bpm, with the initial Hz setting at therapeutic initiation of 5 Hz.[23] The constant mP_{aw} avoids both increases in peak airway pressure and low end-expiratory pressures, decreasing barotrauma. Oscillation contributes to the elimination of CO_2 and reduced trapping of air. Air trapping, also called auto PEEP, is a negative consequence of noncompliant lungs in which a breath is not fully exhaled. Auto PEEP is associated with increased intrathoracic pressure due to an inability to eliminate lung volume during expiration. It produces a stacked-breath pressurized state which leads to a reduction in gas exchange surface area and decrease in cardiac output. In HFOV, the high-frequency oscillation reduces the potential for air trapping and negative consequences of auto PEEP.

HFOV requires specialized ventilators that manipulate specific variables: mean airway pressure measured in cm H_2O, frequency measured in Hz, inspiratory time, and oscillatory pressure amplitude measured in delta power (ΔP) ranging from 1 to 10. Delta power is the pressure amplitude to achieve chest wall vibration.[9] Tidal volume increase is manipulated by decreasing frequency (Hz), increasing ΔP and increasing inspiratory time. This is contrasted to manipulating decreased tidal volume by increasing frequency (Hertz), reducing ΔP, and using shorter inspiratory times. A prominent goal of HFOV management is to maintain ventilation utilizing the highest frequency and the lowest ΔP possible.

Initial settings

Recommendations for initial mPaw settings are increased by 5 cm H_2O from conventional ventilation—consistently noted between 30 and 40 cm H_2O at the beginning of therapy. Newly studied pressure amplitudes range from 60 to 90 cm H_2O.[29] To convey an inspiratory-to-expiratory ratio (I/E) of 1:2, inspiratory time is set at 33%. Oxygenation is maintained by F_iO_2% ranging from 0.6 to 1.0. Ventilation is adjusted by changing the frequency in Hz and ΔP.[23]

Studies that have measured outcomes in lung injury states (ALI and ARDS) have concluded that HFOV is an ideal lung protective MV mode if recruitment efforts are performed.[25] Furthermore, the oscillation frequency and the diameter of the endotracheal (ET) tube may be important variables in the efficacy of ventilation.[26] There have been multiple animal studies that have highlighted the benefits from ventilator induced lung injury (VILI) when HFOV was used.[25] However, further clinical trials and the careful awareness of patient outcomes remain necessary to appreciate this newer mode of ventilation.[25]

HFOV is evolving in its application but is frequently used for patients with significant acute inflammatory pulmonary disease or injury (eg, inhalation injury, influenza). Nursing considerations include the continued assessment of oxygen saturation, arterial blood gases (ABG) analysis, chest radiograph comparisons, and mP_{aw} with ΔP awareness as monitored on the ventilator screens. Traditional MV measurement principles do not apply with HFOV and there is a lack of classic value presence in HFOV; most notably minute ventilation and tidal volume norms. Inspiratory/expiratory auscultatory physical assessments are now challenged owing to oscillatory noise and continual chest movement.

To use this mode in patients with refractory hypoxemia and ventilatory difficulties requires early and aggressive supportive care. As with any newer technology, HFOV clinical exposure and expertise are vital to appropriate clinical usage and management.

Noninvasive Ventilatory Modes

Noninvasive ventilation (NIV), also called noninvasive positive pressure ventilation (NPPV), provides a form of pulmonary support without the risks associated with endotracheal intubation. Increasingly NIV is becoming more common as an effective, early mode of ventilation. Patients with oxygenation and ventilation derangements may benefit from NIV before requiring endotracheal intubation and full MV support.[30] A recent study found that the use of NIV accelerated the improvement in lung function and shortened the critical care and hospital length of stay in asthmatic patients.[31] Primary limitations of NIV are patient selection. The patient must be able to spontaneously breathe, have moderate hemodynamically stability, lack facial or nasal lesions that prevent effective fit of nasal cannula/mask, and cannot have excessive secretions.[30] When implemented early in the management of patients requiring pulmonary support, NIV is a safe and effective noninvasive intervention to improve pulmonary function.[32]

Bilevel positive airway pressure and continuous positive airway pressure

The two most common forms of NIV are bilevel positive airway pressure (BiPAP) and continuous positive airway pressure (CPAP). BiPAP, as the name suggests, employs two cycles of positive pressure to support oxygenation and ventilation. Pressure support is administered to augment inspiration and CPAP to support alveolar opening on expiration.[21,33] With BiPAP the inspiratory pressure is set to achieve optimal tidal volume and CPAP to maximize oxygenation through maintaining open alveoli at end expiration. Adjustments in pressure are made to facilitate ventilation and oxygenation needs for the patient. This mode of therapy is primarily used in instances when gas exchange problems exist and for patients who are spontaneously breathing, but lack signs of respiratory distress. By providing assistance with maintaining alveolar opening, CPAP primarily assists with diffusion of oxygen.

Provided the patient can initiate a spontaneous breath, BiPAP has been found to be effective in supporting a variety of pulmonary disorders (eg, chronic obstructive pulmonary disease [COPD], ARDS/ALI, metabolic acidosis pneumonia, hypoxemia).[30,33] Nursing care priorities in the management of the patient with NIV focus on (1) ensuring optimal mask fit and comfort, (2) tolerance of the NIV mode, (3) assessment of signs of increased work of breathing and fatigue, and (4) effectiveness of the intervention in treating/supporting the respiratory disorder.[21,31,33]

Average volume assured pressure support

Average volume assured pressure support (AVAPS) is a newer mode of NIV that combines both the pressure and volume characteristics of ventilation with a range of inspiratory pressures to guarantee a fixed tidal volume.[34] AVAPS differs from BiPAP in the ability of this mode to ensure more consistent minute ventilation by slowly adjusting inspiratory positive airway pressure to achieve a preset tidal volume.[35] It is a hybrid mode of ventilation that achieves the goal for a given tidal volume with reduced muscle workload. By achieving a consistent tidal volume there is increased consistency in gas exchange. AVAPS has been predominantly used in patients with chronic hypoventilation associated with obesity and sleep apnea.[34,36] Similar to other NIV modes an adequate mask fit is essential for effective therapy. Unique to this mode is the ability to sense changes in tidal volume that allow the NIV to adapt pressure support necessary to meet the goal ventilation predetermined to meet the patient's ventilatory needs. By adapting pressures to ensure goal tidal volume, patient comfort and efficiency in breathing is obtained.[33,36] Care of the patient on AVAPS NIV is similar to that on other modes of NIV.

SUMMARY

Although no single mode of MV has consistently demonstrated superior clinical outcomes, we do know that lung protective strategies that incorporate lower tidal volumes based on IBW have shown a significant reduction in mortality. However, increased sophistication in ventilator technology is providing multiple modes to support the patient during critical illness. Strategies that maximize open lung therapies; limit pressure; and optimize air flow, oxygenation, and ventilation are preferred.[4,8,18,23] Regardless of the mode of MV used, the nurse's knowledge of the mode, monitoring parameters, and intended goals that are to be achieved by the mode are essential in the requisite care of critically ill patients. Nurses are well positioned to monitor MV effectiveness and provide assessment data concerning the success of this lifesaving intervention for the critical care team.

Partnered appreciation of lung protective strategies in critical care includes evidence critique by physicians, nurses, and respiratory therapists. Further inquiry and research are also necessary for both present and future modes of MV. An effective care strategy encompasses active dialogue regarding current evidence, assessment considerations, clinical recommendations, acknowledgment of patient complexities, and a dynamic evaluative approach. Patients depend on this active collaboration at their most vulnerable phases of critical illness.

REFERENCES

1. Gajic O, Saquib I, Mendez J, et al. Ventilator-associated lung injury in patients without acute lung injury at the onset of mechanical ventilation. Crit Care Med 2004;32(9): 1817–24.
2. Orlando R. Ventilators: how clever, how complex? [editorial]. Crit Care Med 2003: 2704–5.
3. Caples M, Hubmayr RD. Respiratory system mechanics and respiratory muscle function. In: Fink MP, Vincent JL, Kochanek, P, editors. Textbook of critical care. 5th edition. Philadelphia: Elsevier Saunders; 2005. p. 473.
4. Haas CR. Mechanical ventilation with lung protective strategies: what works? Crit Care Clin 2011;27(3):469–86.
5. Challuri L. Acute respiratory failure. In: Fink MP, Vincent JL, Kochanek, P, editors. Textbook of critical care. 5th edition. Philadelphia: Elsevier Saunders; 2005. p. 39.
6. Lachmann B. Open up the lung and keep the lung open. Intensive Care Med 1992; 18(6):319–21.
7. Papadkos PJ, Lachmann B. The open lung concept of alveolar recruitment can improve outcomes in respiratory failure and ARDS. Mt Sinai J Med 2002; 69(1):73–7.

8. Gattinoni L, Carlesso EI, Caironi P. Stress and strain within the lung. Curr Opin Crit Care 2012;18(1):42–7.

9. Burns S. Pressure modes of mechanical ventilation: the good, the bad, and the ugly. AACN Adv Crit Care 2008;19(4):399–411.

10. Gattinoni L, Protti AI, Caironi P, et al. Ventilator-induced lung injury: the anatomical and physiological framework. Crit Care Med 2010;39(10):S539–48.

11. Kumar A, Pontoppidan H, Falke KJ, et al. Pulmonary barotrauma during mechanical ventilation. Crit Care Med 1973;1(1):181–6.

12. Dos Santos CC, Slutsky AS. Mechanisms of ventilator-induced lung injury: a perspective. J Appl Physiol 2000;89(4):1645–55.

13. Burns S. Invasive mechanical ventilation (through an artificial airway): volume and pressure modes and indices of oxygenation. In: Weigand D. editor. AACN procedure manual for critical care. 6th edition. Philadelphia: Elsevier Saunders; 2011. p. 262–84.

14. Meade MO, Cook DJ, Guyatt GH, et al and Lung Open Ventilation Study Investigators. Ventilation strategy using low tidal volumes, recruitment maneuvers, and high positive end-expiratory pressure for acute lung injury and acute respiratory distress syndrome: a randomized controlled trial. JAMA 2008;299(6):637–45.

15. NIH NHLBI ARDS Clinical Network. Available at: http://www.ardsnet.org/system/files/Ventilator%20Protocol%20Card.pdf. Accessed March 31, 2012.

16. Brower RG, Matthay MA, Morris A, et al. Ventilation with lower tidal volumes as compared with traditional tidal volumes for acute lung injury and the acute respiratory distress syndrome. N Engl J Med 2000;342(18):1301–8.

17. Esan A, Hess D, Raoof S, et al. Severe hypoxemic respiratory failure part 1—ventilatory strategies. Chest 2010;137(5):1203–13.

18. Determann R, Royakkers A, Wolthuis E, et al. Ventilation with lower tidal volumes as compared with conventional tidal volumes for patients without acute lung injury: a preventive randomized controlled trial. Crit Care Med 2010;14:R1.

19. Habashi N. Other approaches to open-lung ventilation: airway pressure release ventilation. Crit Care Med 2005;33(3 Suppl):228–40.

20. Estaban A, Alia I, Gordo F, et al. Prospective randomized trial comparing pressure controlled ventilation and volume controlled ventilation in ARDS. Chest 2000;117(6): 1690–6.

21. Cawley MJ. Mechanical ventilation: introduction for the pharmacy practitioner. J Pharm Pract 2011;24(1):7–16.

22. Singer B, Corbridge T. Pressure modes of invasive mechanical ventilation. Southern Med J 2011;104(10):701–9.

23. Rose L. Advanced modes of mechanical ventilation: implications for practice. AACN Adv Crit Care 2006;17(2):145–60.

24. Bosma K, Ferreyra G, Ambrogio C, et al. Patient ventilator interaction and sleep in mechanically ventilated patients: pressure support versus proportional assist ventilation. Crit Care Med 2007;35(4):1048–54.

25. Imai Y, Slutsky AS. High frequency oscillatory ventilation and ventilator-induced lung injury. Crit Care Med 2005;33(3 Suppl):S129–34.

26. Hager DN, Fessler HE, Kaczka DW, et al. Tidal volume delivery during high-frequency oscillatory ventilation in adults with acute respiratory distress syndrome. Crit Care Med 2007;35(6):1522–9.

27. Derdak S, Mehta S, Stewart T, et al. High frequency oscillatory ventilation for acute respiratory distress syndrome in adults: a randomized, controlled trial. Am J Respir Crit Care Med 2002;166:801–8.

28. Mehta S, Granton J, MacDonald R, et al. High-frequency oscillatory ventilation in adults: the Toronto experience. Chest 2004;126(2):518–27.

29. Derdak S. Lung-protective higher frequency oscillatory ventilation. Crit Care Med 2008;36(4):1358–9.
30. Boldrini R, Fasano L, Stefano N. Noninvasive mechanical ventilation. Curr Opin Crit Care 2012;18(10):48–53.
31. Gupta D, Nath A, Agarwal R, et al. A prospective randomized controlled trial on the efficacy of noninvasive ventilation in severe acute asthma. Respir Care 2010;55(5): 536–43.
32. Burns KE, Adhikari NK, Keenan SP, et al. Use of noninvasive ventilation to wean critically ill adults off invasive ventilation: meta-analysis and systematic review. Br Med J 2009;338(5):1574–80.
33. Hill NS, Brennan J, Garpestad E, et al. Noninvasive ventilation in acute respiratory failure. Crit Care Med 2007;35(10):2402–7.
34. Crisafulli E, Manni G, Kidonias M., et al. Subjective sleep quality during average volume assured pressure support ventilation in patients with hypercapnic COPD: a physiological pilot study. Lung 2009;187;299–305.
35. Roussos M, Parthasarathy S, Ayas NT. Can we improve sleep quality by changing the way we ventilate patients? Lung 2010;188:1–3.
36. Storre JH, Seuthe B, Fiechter R, et al. Average volume assured pressure support in obesity hypoventilation: a randomized crossover trial. Chest 139(3):815–21.

Weaning from Mechanical Ventilation
Where Were We Then, and Where Are We Now?

Suzanne M. Burns, MSN, RRT, ACNP, CCRN, FCCM

KEYWORDS

- Weaning from mechanical ventilation • Ventilator weaning • Ventilator liberation
- Weaning protocols • Weaning guidelines • Sedation management

KEY POINTS

- Gains have been made in selected outcomes such as ventilator duration, but key metrics such as hospital length of stay and mortality are still not optimum despite randomized controlled trials that define how best to initiate management strategies such as weaning trials (ie, weaning screens and spontaneous breathing trials), sedation interruptions, and prophylaxis interventions to prevent hospital-associated complications.
- Adherence to protocols and guidelines derived from even the best studies is poor in part because they add complexity to the bedside.
- These clinical tools should be carefully applied and/or adapted for practical use before implementation.

Weaning patients from long-term mechanical ventilation (LTMV) has been an important focus of clinical process improvement initiatives and research for decades. Because extended durations of ventilation are associated with negative clinical and institutional outcomes, we continue to look for methods that hasten ventilator liberation, especially for those who require prolonged ventilation (≥72 hours). Although numerous studies have suggested that the weaning process is greatly facilitated with protocols and guidelines for weaning trials and sedation management,[1–7] outcomes for this population of patients continues to be less than desirable. For example, the mortality of patients ventilated for greater than 96 hours and those ventilated less than 96 hours in the United States is cited to be 34% versus 35% respectively with a combined annual aggregated hospital cost of less than $16 billion.[8]

Clinicians who manage or care for ventilated patients work to ensure that care is evidence-based by using protocols and guidelines derived from randomized controlled

The author is the inventor of the Burns Wean Assessment Program (BWAP) and holds the copyright.
University of Virginia Health System, School of Nursing, University of Virginia, Box 800826, Claude Moore Building, 225 Jeanette Lancaster Way, Charlottesville, VA 22903-3387, USA
E-mail address: smb4h@virginia.edu

trials (RCTs). Findings from these studies suggest that the use of protocols and guidelines result in improved outcomes such as shorter intensive care unit (ICU) and hospital lengths of stay (LOS), lower mortality, and lower costs.[1–7] Unfortunately, studies note that when research protocols and guidelines are applied to practice, adherence may be poor.[9–19] This has led some to suggest that we need to make a "mid-course correction" in the way we do things.[20] To that end, considering where we have been and where we are now with weaning practices may be a first step.

The purpose of this article is to describe the science that drives our current weaning practices, including (1) pre-weaning assessment, (2) individualized weaning plans, (3) weaning prediction, (4) the use of protocols and guidelines for weaning trials and sedation management, (5) timing of tracheostomy placement, and (6) system initiatives for the management of LTMV patients. Finally, this article discusses potential interventions for improving the outcomes of patients who require prolonged mechanical ventilation.

WEANING: SCIENCE AND PRACTICE
Weaning Predictors

In the 1980s, weaning from long-term mechanical ventilation was an arduous process. Individualized plans for improving the patients' overall physical state during the pre-weaning stage (ie, the patient is stable yet numerous clinical impediments to active weaning exist) were the norm, with little standardization. Determination of weaning readiness was often accomplished by testing the patient with various weaning predictors such as standard weaning parameters (ie, negative inspiratory pressure, positive expiratory pressure, spontaneous tidal volume, and vital capacity), the rapid-shallow breathing index (f_x/V_t), the wean index (WI), and occlusion pressure (P.01) to name just a few.[21–24] Despite early study outcomes that suggested the predictors reliably identified the ability of the patient to be successfully extubated, their use in practice and subsequent studies suggested that they were not reliable positive predictors, that is, they did not tell us when the patient *could* wean.[25,26] In addition, the predictors tested pulmonary factors to the exclusion of nonpulmonary factors for readiness to wean. Their use diminished except as a means of predicting weaning failure (ie, as negative predictors), and to that end, some have been used in current studies to do just that. One recent study used a threshold number for the f_x/V_t as a criterion for application of the "wake up and breathe" study protocol.[7] The use of weaning predictors to date is rare except in examples such as noted in the Girard study.[7] This is in large part due to the positive results of studies accomplished in the late 1990s that focused on weaning methods, specifically the use of weaning protocols and guidelines for sedation management.

Protocols and Guidelines for Weaning Trials and Sedation Management

The use of protocols for weaning trials was stimulated by the work of Brochard and colleagues and Esteban and colleagues, in RCTs testing the efficacy of different modes of ventilation applied by protocol to patients requiring prolonged ventilation.[27,28] The results of these two studies were similar in that they both demonstrated that weaning protocols, regardless of the ventilator mode, resulted in shorter ventilator duration than when weaning was accomplished via the existing "standard" (ie, individually tailored wean plan). In the Esteban study, patients (n = 546) who met study criteria were placed on a spontaneous breathing trial (SBT) for 2 hours.[28] If the patient did not tolerate the trial he or she was randomly assigned to a specific weaning protocol (ie, intermittent mandatory ventilation [IMV], pressure support ventilation [PSV], or SBT) or the control method (ie, standard weaning method). If the patient passed the 2-hour SBT he or she was extubated; 20% of these patients required reintubation.[28] Ely and colleagues tested the safety and efficacy of a SBT as described by Esteban.[1] The study used a weaning screen to identify stability (eg, a series of clinical markers such as breathing rate, oxygenation, and hemodynamic status) followed by a 2-hour SBT if the criteria were met. The study took place in medical and coronary care units. The process was found to be both safe and effective. Positive outcomes included shorter ventilator duration (4.5 vs 6 days, $P = .003$) and fewer complications such as reintubation and need for tracheostomy in the intervention versus control groups (20% vs 41% respectively, $P = .001$). These studies also demonstrated the efficacy of using health care providers such as nurses and respiratory therapists to apply the protocols.[1,2,5,29–31] The positive outcomes, plus the ease of use and efficiency of the SBT protocols, were attractive to clinicians. After publication of these studies, many hospitals sought similar outcomes by applying the protocols to practice.

But, despite gains in shortening ventilator duration in some patients by standardizing the process of weaning trials, other outcomes such as ICU and hospital LOS (as noted earlier) were still not optimal.[1,2,5] A potential aspect of care, specifically the use of sedation infusions, was forwarded as a potential culprit of delayed weaning in a study by Kollef and colleagues.[2] Although the primary goal of the study was to test the efficacy of a weaning method using a nurse/therapist driven weaning protocol, the authors noted a relationship between delayed weaning and sedation infusion use.[2] Subsequently Brook and colleagues performed an RCT, testing the efficacy of a nurse-driven sedation management algorithm compared to standard management.[3] Their findings noted that the algorithmic approach resulted in a significantly shorter ICU LOS (5.7 vs 7.5 days respectively, $P = .013$) and hospital LOS (14 vs 19 days respectively, $P<.001$).[3] To explore this association further, Kress and colleagues conducted an RCT to compare daily sedation interruptions to standard sedation management and found that the interruption method decreased duration of ventilation (4.9 vs 7.3 days respectively, $P = .004$) and ICU LOS (6.4 vs 9.9 days respectively, $P = .02$).[4] In another study using the same database, the investigators found that patients in the "interruption" group experienced fewer complications as compared to the conventional sedation management group (2.8% vs 6.2% complications, $P = .04$).[6]

But all were not comfortable with the process of withdrawing sedative agents. Concerns emerged related to the potential psychological harm imposed by the abrupt withdrawal of the drugs. To that end, the authors sought to determine the effect of the sedation interruptions on the patients who had been enrolled in the daily sedation interruption study.[32] Using a battery of psychological tests, the authors found that those who experienced the daily interruptions experienced either a significant decrease in psychological stress or equivalent stress ("Total Impact of Events Score" 11.2 vs 27.3, $P = .02$; "Incidence of PTSD" 0 vs 3.2%, $P = .06$; and "Psychosocial Adjustment to Illness Score" 46.8 vs 54.3, $P = .08$), to those who were cared for in a traditional manner (ie, slower, gradual sedation withdrawal).[32] Finally, in another RCT referred to as the "wake up and breathe" trial, Girard and colleagues paired a sedation interruption with a SBT and found that the paired intervention resulted in increased ventilator-free days (group: 14.7 vs 11.6, $P = .02$), shorter time to discharge from the ICU and hospital (ICU days: 9.1 vs 12.9, $P = .01$; hospital days: 14.9 vs 19.2, $P = .04$), and better 1-year mortality (44% vs 58%) than those in the control group.[7]

Although the association between weaning outcomes and sedation was noted and addressed in the described studies, an additional concern related to outcomes of ventilated patients surrounds the relationship of sedative use (especially benzodiazepines) to delirium and long-term cognitive dysfunction.[33-37] In a study of 224 ventilated coronary care and medical intensive care patients Ely and colleagues found that up to 81% of the mechanically ventilated patients experienced delirium.[35,36] Patients with delirium experienced higher 6-month mortality rates (34% vs 15%, $P = .03$) and spent 10 days longer in the hospital than those who never developed delirium ($P<.001$). Because sedation is commonly used in critical care to assist with stabilization and management of ventilated patients, and is associated with many complications (eg, delayed weaning, longer ICU and hospital LOSs, and the development of delirium), it is clear that sedation management is a key aspect of care for ventilated patients and must be part of what we do.

Unfortunately, the use of sedation is complex. Studies exploring the use of the protocols and guidelines (these terms are often used interchangeably) report that adherence to the described protocols is very poor.[9-19] Although most of the studies on adherence to sedation interruption have been done using survey methodology, the results are compelling and suggest multiple reasons for the lack of adherence. As described in a review of the literature by the author of this article, reasons include caregiver perceptions (eg, that amnesia is good for patients, that it is unsafe to remove sedatives abruptly), the complexity associated with using protocols and guidelines (eg, multiple steps and the inherent "take-it-or-leave it" nature of guideline recommendations), and the philosophy and care practices of the environment in which they are implemented.[38] Examples of the latter include a series of studies conducted in Australian ICUs, where the nurses' practices incorporated their philosophy that sedatives must be used sparingly.[39-41] When these nurses tested outcomes associated with their accepted sedation management practices as compared to using sedation guidelines or other related tools such as sedation scales, they found the use of the tools to be redundant, ineffective, and potentially harmful.[39-41] For example, in the study by Elliott and colleagues, the use of a sedation algorithm resulted in slower sedation removal and an increase in ventilator duration (4.8 days preintervention vs 5.6 days postintervention [NS]) and LOS (7.1 days preintervention vs 8.2 days postintervention ($P = .04$).[39] These authors also found that patients assigned to the algorithm were more sedated than those not assigned (NS).[39] Williams and colleagues found that the addition of sedation scales delayed sedation withdrawal, and Bucknall and colleagues noted that use of a sedation protocol made no difference in duration of ventilation or ICU and hospital LOS.[40,41]

It may be that our lack of progress in attaining desired weaning outcomes is due to poor translation of research to practice; that protocols are not designed well for clinical use. And, if we are not adhering to the protocols, we cannot expect to have the same desired weaning outcomes as described in the studies. So although the use of protocols and guidelines for weaning trials and sedation management has the potential for improving outcomes of mechanical ventilation, we have a way to go to ensure that what we "think" we are doing is actually what we are doing. Other aspects of care may also contribute to the outcomes of interest and should be considered. They include clinical factors that positively or negatively affect weaning potential and timing of tracheostomy placement.

Pre-Weaning Assessments of Clinical Factors That Affect Weaning Potential

Patients who require prolonged mechanical ventilation (>72 hours) suffer from a myriad of conditions and diagnoses that complicate their ability to breathe spontaneously. A consensus document on weaning was published in 2001 that recommended that active weaning trials should occur when clinical factors and conditions that adversely affect the patients' weaning potential are corrected before attempting

Patient _____

Yes/ No/ Not assessed   **GENERAL ASSESSMENT**

___   ___   ___   1. Hemodynamically stable (pulse rate, cardiac output)?

___   ___   ___   2. Free from factors that increase or decrease metabolic rate (seizures, temperature, sepsis, bacteremia, hypo/hyperthyroid)?

___   ___   ___   3. Hematocrit >25% (or baseline)?

___   ___   ___   4. Systemically hydrated (weight at or near baseline, balanced intake and output)?

___   ___   ___   5. Nourished (albumin >2.5, parenteral/enteral feedings maximized)? (If albumin is low and anasarca or third spacing is present, score for hydration should be No.)

___   ___   ___   6. Electrolytes with in normal limits? (including Ca^{2+}, Mg^{2+}, HPO_4^{2-}).

                     *Correct Ca^{2+} for albumin level.

___   ___   ___   7. Pain controlled? (subjective determination)

___   ___   ___   8. Adequate sleep/rest ? (subjective determination)

___   ___   ___   9. Appropriate level of anxiety and nervousness? (subjective determination)

___   ___   ___   10. Absence of bowel problems (diarrhea, constipation, ileus)?

___   ___   ___   11. Improved general body strength and endurance (eg, out of bed in chair, progressive activity program)?

___   ___   ___   12. Chest x-ray improving?

Respiratory Assessment

Gas flow and work of breathing

___   ___   ___   13. Eupneic respiratory rate and pattern (spontaneous respiratory rate <25, without dyspnea, absence of accessory muscle use).

                     *This is assessed off the ventilator while measuring #20-23.

___   ___   ___   14. Absence of adventitious breath sounds (rhonchi, rales, wheezing)?

___   ___   ___   15. Secretions thin and minimal?

___   ___   ___   16. Absence of neuromuscular disease/deformity?

___   ___   ___   17. Absence of abdominal distention/obesity/ascites?

___   ___   ___   18. Oral endotracheal tube ≥ 7.5 or trach ≥ 6.5

Airway clearance

___   ___   ___   19. Cough and swallow reflexes adequate?

Strength

___   ___   ___   20. Negative inspiratory pressure <-20 cm H2O

___   ___   ___   21. Positive expiratory pressure >+30 cm H2O

Endurance

___   ___   ___   22. Spontaneous tidal volume >5 mL/kg?

___   ___   ___   23. Vital capacity >10 to 15 mL/kg?

Arterial blood gases

___   ___   ___   24. pH between 7.30 - 7.45

___   ___   ___   25. $PaCO_2$ approximately 40 mm Hg (or baseline) with minute ventilation <10 L/min (evaluated while on ventilator)

___   ___   ___   26. PaO_2 >60 on FiO_2 <40%

To score the BWAP: divide the number of "yes" responses by 26

Fig. 1. Burns Wean Assessment Program Worksheet. (© 1990, S.M. Burns.)

weaning and extubation.[42] Although this seems a logical first step, there have been few tools developed to ensure that a comprehensive approach occurs.

One comprehensive pre-weaning checklist, the Burns Wean Assessment Program (BWAP), was specifically designed to assist the clinician in systematically assessing 26 clinical factors that may impede weaning in patients requiring long-term mechanical ventilation[26,43,44] (**Fig. 1**). In a series of studies describing an institutional approach to weaning using advanced practice nurses as "Outcomes Managers," the BWAP was used as a checklist to efficiently focus on factors needing correction before conducting a weaning trial.[29–31] The checklist was used routinely as part a clinical system initiative designed to monitor and manage patients requiring ventilation for greater than 72 hours in five adult critical care units.[30,31] Outcomes such as ventilator duration, ICU and hospital LOS, and mortality met or exceeded national benchmarks during the 7 year tenure of the program. Subsequent studies also noted the use of the BWAP as a predictor of weaning potential and described the importance of the individual factors to weaning outcomes.[43,44] Perhaps most importantly, the work using the BWAP suggested that regardless of where the patient originated (eg, neurologic vs medical unit vs surgical unit), patients who require mechanical ventilation for greater than 3 days are more similar than different.[43,44] For example, with delayed weaning, the original problem that necessitated mechanical ventilation may be less responsible for the inability to wean than iatrogenic conditions that emerge over time, such as bloodstream infection, sepsis, deep vein thrombosis, pulmonary embolus, hyperglycemia, ventilator-associated pneumonia, urinary tract infection, and immobility. Thus, it is reasonable to assume that one of the steps in weaning consist of a comprehensive, systematic approach that addresses the many factors that potentially impede weaning progress in all patient categories. Although most multidisciplinary teams assume that this is done routinely in daily rounds, it may not be. In part this unintended variation in practice is why a clinical checklist like the BWAP is an important tool to improve outcomes. Its use should be encouraged.[45]

Timing of Tracheostomy

In the past, the role of a tracheostomy in weaning patients requiring prolonged ventilation was unclear with the exception of those patients with conditions for which the need for tracheostomy is obvious early in the admission (eg, those with spinal cord injury and paralysis). For others, the placement and timing of tracheostomy was generally accomplished when repeated attempts at weaning were unsuccessful and the endotracheal tube was impeding other functions such as mobilization, eating, and talking. Although "time to tracheostomy" has decreased over the years from about 21 to 12 days (personal communications of the author with numerous health care facilities), there continues to be numerous opinions related to the relationship of timing of tracheostomy to clinical outcomes. Unfortunately, few studies have been performed to test these relationships. Some exceptions exist and brief descriptions follow.

Studies on the timing of tracheostomy suggest that early versus late tracheostomy placement (terms vary with the studies) is beneficial for the patient and improves selected outcomes. In an observational study by Brook and colleagues, early tracheostomy was associated with shorter duration of ventilation (28.3 vs 34.4 days in the early vs late tracheostomy placement, $P = .005$) and hospital cost ($86,189 vs $124,649, $P = .001$) in medical ICU patients.[46] In a retrospective review, Freeman and colleagues found that earlier timing of tracheostomy was associated with shorter ventilator duration and ICU and hospital LOS ($r = .341$, $P<.001$ for all).[47] In another observational study (n = 312), Nieszkowska and colleagues noted that patients who receive a tracheostomy actually require less sedation, spend less time heavily sedated, and achieve autonomy earlier than those who do not receive a tracheostomy.[48] Finally, Rumback and colleagues conducted a prospective RCT comparing early percutaneous dilational tracheotomy to prolonged translaryngeal intubation (delayed tracheotomy) in critically ill medical patients.[49] In this study, 120 patients projected to require mechanical ventilation for greater than 14 days were randomly assigned to percutaneous tracheostomy within 48 hours. Mortality, pneumonia, and accidental extubations were all statistically significantly improved in the early tracheostomy group as compared to the delayed tracheostomy group (mortality: 31.7% vs 61.7%; pneumonia: 5% vs 25%; and accidental extubations: 0 vs 6 respectively). In addition, the early tracheostomy patients had shorter ICU LOS (4.8 vs 16.2 days), shorter ventilator duration (7.6 vs 17.4 days), and less damage to the mouth and larynx than those assigned to the control group (ie, surgical tracheostomy when determined appropriate by the health care team.[49]

These findings suggest that early tracheostomy is conducive to earlier weaning as well as other desirable outcomes. However, assigning patients to tracheostomy within 48 hours is unlikely to be applied as a standard management step in the care of these patients. Regardless, it is important to consider the results of the Rumback study in conjunction with that of the findings of Nieszkowska and colleagues. It may be that by placing a tracheostomy earlier, less sedative use is necessary and outcomes are improved. To attain good outcomes in these patients, clinicians charged with their care should consider early tracheostomy placement. This may be especially important if practice patterns do not ensure regular attempts to discontinue sedatives!

Comprehensive, Systematic Approaches to the Care of LTMV Patients

Weaning patients is not simply about the ventilator, but instead about the myriad of conditions and clinical factors that impede weaning progress. Thus, the answer to the question "how best to wean our patients?" is not an easy or singular one such as to employ a weaning trial protocol. Instead the complexity of these patients demands a more comprehensive, systematic, and perhaps more labor-intensive method.

System initiatives that incorporate numerous evidence-based elements of care, such as those addressed earlier, into a formalized approach for the LTMV patient are focused on decreasing practice variation.[29–31,50] Evidence-based clinical pathways may be used to clarify when to initiate selected care elements such as nutrition, mobility, tracheostomy placement, weaning trials, and prophylaxis (eg, for gastrointestinal bleeding, deep vein thrombosis, sinusitis, glucose control, and sedation management). Importantly, clinicians (often advanced practice nurses called outcomes managers) are identified to manage the process, coordinate the multidisciplinary approach, and monitor the outcomes.[29–31,50] Although labor intensive to initiate and sustain, the programs report positive clinical and financial outcomes and they assure that sustained attention to monitoring and managing the processes of care occurs.[29–31,50] This is an important aspect of this type of care management initiative as the inherent complexity of protocols and guidelines make it unlikely that adherence will be good without rigorous attention. And, as noted previously, lack of adherence may result in unintended consequences.[38] For example, in a study by Girard and colleagues, a sedation interruption was paired with an SBT.[7] Although this pairing on face value appears sensible and straightforward, it is rarely so. In the study, the steps are monitored and managed as part of a research protocol with all the attendant safeguards (and personnel) to ensure adherence. When used as part of a bedside care guideline, separate from the rigor assured in a scientific study, the guideline steps are unlikely to be accomplished as designed. Further, the forced focus on the guideline steps may put nurses and other care givers "off their game" as they focus on the often complicated steps of the guidelines versus other key aspects of care. Although the development of system initiatives such as described may be difficult to design and sustain, associated outcomes make them attractive options for the current complex health care system to embrace.

SO WHERE ARE WE NOW ... WHAT SHOULD WE DO TO ASSURE GOOD OUTCOMES FOR OUR PATIENTS?

Given where we have been, and what we have learned to date about weaning patients from LTMV, the following elements should be considered for incorporation into programs for the management of this patient population.

Use a Comprehensive Method for Assessing the Patients' Physical Progress or Lack Thereof

The BWAP has been used successfully in the author's institution to ensure that care elements listed in the checklist are addressed appropriately and in a timely manner while considering process factors that may take precedence.[30,31] Whether or not this tool is used as a clinical checklist or not, a method of systematically assessing key care elements is essential. And, if factors that impede weaning are present, interventions to address these should be initiated. It is helpful to have the care elements delineated in terms of best-practice and the appropriate interventions accepted by key clinical stakeholders so that team "buy-in" is high and adherence more likely. For example, although the use of progressive activity or mobility programs appears to be associated with good outcomes in patients requiring LTMV,[51–54] a mobility program should be established that is reasonable and practical in terms of application within an ICU setting.

Apply Evidence-Based Protocols and Guidelines Carefully

Although there is little controversy related to the importance of using evidence-based protocols for weaning trials and sedation withdrawal, how we use them should be carefully considered. SBTs are relatively straightforward but the trial timing and duration may be an issue to address because competing care elements may offset the potential effectiveness of the trials. This is especially true if using the paired sedation withdrawal and SBT protocol (ie, "wake up and breathe"). Ensure that caregivers are able to spend the time required to monitor and manage the protocol elements when they are initiated or the outcomes may not be positive.

The importance of sedation withdrawal cannot be overstated. Long-term use of sedatives is to be discouraged except when absolutely necessary. Unfortunately, the use of sedatives is still erroneously considered necessary for comfort and to ensure amnesia,[17] despite data that links the use of the drugs to delirium, long-term cognitive dysfunction, and other negative outcomes.[33–37] Perhaps the best way to ensure that sedation withdrawal occurs is to discourage the routine use of the drugs in tandem with analgesics. Pain management is an essential part of care and delivery of the drugs is best done in a manner to ensure a steady state. This is not true of sedatives except when used in the operating room, for short-term procedural use, and when paralytic agents are necessary. In other cases, the ordering of the drugs as an infusion should be discouraged in favor of bolus or enteral sedatives. As noted in a RCT by Strom and colleagues, the use of a protocol of no sedation in mechanically ventilated patients resulted in better outcomes than when sedation was used.[55] Education of clinicians about the untoward effects of sedatives in these patients is an important first step but in addition, processes that make it easy to do the right thing are essential.

Consider Early Versus Late Tracheostomy

Early tracheostomy may result in better outcomes including mortality.[49] However, few will likely integrate early tracheostomy (on day 2) into weaning programs. Regardless, if adherence to sedation management withdrawal continues to be a problem, it seems that early tracheostomy may be an essential care element.

Manage and Monitor Outcomes of Weaning Initiatives

Many clinical outcomes are monitored by regulatory agencies to compare differences between like institutions. While important, key metrics are as yet not monitored by individual institutions and should be. One example is adherence to protocols and guidelines. As described previously, although a protocol or guideline may be in place, adherence is not assured. And if adherence is not good, then how can outcomes be related to their use? A key metric that is unfortunately not routinely monitored is that of extubation (planned and unplanned). Although SBTs and subsequent extubation efforts are designed to liberate patients as efficiently and effectively as possible, extubation outcomes are not always monitored. In a study by Thille and colleagues, outcomes of extubation failure in medical intensive care unit patients were associated with marked deterioration in clinical status.[56] Although we do not wish to unduly extend intubation time needlessly, overzealous and/or inappropriately premature extubations are risky. Premature attempts may result in the need for reintubation and potentially poor outcomes, yet delayed extubations are equally dangerous because hospital-acquired conditions may ensue. Although no data to date have emerged that identify an appropriate reintubation rate after extubation attempts; one study suggests that a failed planned extubation rate of 9% to 15% is associated with more ventilator and ICU-free days than when the rates were either higher or lower (Kapnadak and colleagues, unpublished data, 2011). Regardless, interventions designed to wean patients should be tracked and evaluated in context with the aggressiveness of the weaning plans. If we do not do so then we do not know what we are doing!

SUMMARY

A panacea for weaning patients from LTMV does not exist. Although gains have been made in selected outcomes such as ventilator duration, key metrics such as hospital LOS and mortality are still not optimum despite RCTs that define how best to initiate management strategies such as weaning trials (ie, weaning screens and SBTs), sedation interruptions, and prophylaxis interventions to prevent hospital-associated complications.

Adherence to protocols and guidelines derived from even the best studies is poor in part because they add complexity to the bedside. These clinical tools should be carefully applied and/or adapted for practical use before implementation. LTMV patients suffer from a myriad of conditions that prevent weaning; our approach of necessity must be both systematic and comprehensive. To do less belies our understanding of them and we will continue to apply protocols and guidelines from studies that address one or two elements of care while diverting a more comprehensive seamless approach. Finally, managing and monitoring what we do for our patients and the related outcomes is essential if we are to determine what works best.

REFERENCES

1. Ely EW, Baker AM, Dunagan DP, et al. Effect on the duration of mechanical ventilation of identifying patients capable of breathing spontaneously. N Engl J Med 1996;335: 1964–9.
2. Kollef MH, Shapiro SD, Silver P, et al. A randomized, controlled trial of protocol-directed versus physician-directed weaning from mechanical ventilation. Crit Care Med 1997;25:567–4.
3. Brook AD, Ahrens TS, Schaff R, et al. Effect of a nursing-implemented sedation protocol on the duration of mechanical ventilation. Crit Care Med 1999;27:2609–15.
4. Kress JP, Pohlman AS, O'Connor MF, et al. Daily interruption of sedative infusions in critically ill patients undergoing mechanical ventilation. N Engl J Med 2000;342: 1471–7.

5. Marelich GP, Murin S, Battistella F, et al. Protocol weaning of mechanical ventilation in medical and surgical patients by respiratory care practitioners and nurses: effect on weaning time and incidence of ventilator associated pneumonia. Chest 2000;118:459–67.
6. Schweickert WD, Gehlbach BK, Pohlman AS, et al. Daily interruptions of sedative infusions and complications of critical illness in mechanically ventilated patients. Crit Care Med 2004;32:1272–6.
7. Girard T, Kress J, Fuchs B, et al. Efficacy and safety of a paired sedation and ventilator weaning protocol for mechanically ventilated patients in intensive care (Awakening and Breathing Controlled trial): a randomised controlled trial. Lancet 2008;371:126–34.
8. Zilberberg MD, Luippold RS, Sulsky S, et al. Prolonged acute mechanical ventilation, hospital resource utilization, and mortality in the United States. Crit Care Med 2008;36;724–30.
9. Bair N, Bobek MB, Hoffman-Hog L, et al. Introduction of sedative, analgesic and neuromuscular blocking agent guidelines in a medical intensive care unit: physician and nurse adherence. Crit Care Med 2000;28:707–13.
10. Botha J, LeBlanc V. The state of sedation in the nation: results of an Australian survey. Crit Care Resuscit 2005;7(2):92–6.
11. Egerod I, Christensen BV, Johansen L. Trends in sedation practices in Danish intensive care units in 2003: a national survey. Intensive Care Med 2006;32:60–6.
12. Martin J, Franck M, Sigel S, et al. Changes in sedation management in German intensive care units between 2002 and 2006: a national follow-up survey. Crit Care 2007;11:R124.
13. Guttormson JL, Chlan L, Weinert C, et al. Factors influencing nurse sedation practices with mechanically ventilated patients: a U.S. national survey. Intensive Crit Care Nurs 2010;26:44–50.
14. Metha S, Burry L, Fischer S, et al; Canadian Critical Care Trials Group. Canadian survey of the use of sedatives, analgesics and neuromuscular blocking agents in critically ill patients. Crit Care Med 2006;34:556–7.
15. Rhoney DH, Murry KR. National survey of the use of sedating drugs, neuromuscular blocking agents, and reversal agents in the intensive care unit. J Intensive Care Med 2003;18:139–45.
16. Samuelson KA, Larson S, Lundberg D, et al. Intensive care sedation of mechanically ventilated patients: a national Swedish survey. Intensive Crit Care Nurs 2003;19:350–62.
17. Slomka J, Hoffman-Hogg L, Mion LC, et al. Influence of clinicians' values and perceptions on use of clinical practice guidelines for sedation and neuromuscular blockade in patients receiving mechanical ventilation. Am J Crit Care 2000;9:412–8.
18. Tanios MA, deWit M, Epstein S, et al. Perceived barriers to the use of sedation protocols and daily sedation interruption: a multidisciplinary survey. J Crit Care 2009;24:66–73.
19. Patel RP, Gambrell M, Speroff T, et al. Delirium and sedation in the intensive care unit: survey of behaviors and attitudes of 1384 healthcare professionals. Crit Care Med 2009;37:825–32.
20. Walker S, Brett S. Oiling the wheels of intensive care to reduce "machine friction": the best way to improve outcomes? Crit Care Med 2010;38(Suppl 10):S642–8.
21. Sahn SA, Lakshimnarayan S, Petty TL. Weaning from mechanical ventilation. JAMA 1976;235:2208–12.
22. Yang K, Tobin MJ. A prospective study of indexes predicting the outcome of trials of weaning from mechanical ventilation. N Engl J Med 1991;324:1445–50.
23. Jabour ER, Rabil DM, Truwit JD, et al. Evaluation of a new weaning index based on ventilatory endurance and the efficiency of gas exchange. Am Rev Respir Dis 1991;144:531–7.

24. Sassoon CS, Te TT, Mahutte CK, et al. An important indicator for successful weaning in patients with chronic obstructive pulmonary disease. Am Rev Respir Dis 1987; 135(1):107–13.
25. Lee KH, Hui KP, Chan TB, et al. Rapid shallow breathing (frequency-tidal volume ratio) did not predict extubation outcome. Chest 1994;105:540–3.
26. Burns SM, Burns JE, Truwit JD. Comparison of five clinical weaning indices. Am J Crit Care 1994;3(5):342–52.
27. Brochard L, Ranes A, Benito S, et al. Comparison of three methods of gradual withdrawal from ventilatory support during weaning from mechanical ventilators. Am Respir Crit Care Med 1994;150:896–903.
28. Esteban A, Frutos F, Tobin MJ, et al. A comparison of four methods of weaning patients from mechanical ventilation. N Engl J Med 1995;332:345–50.
29. Burns SM, Marshall M, Burns JE, et al. Design, testing and outcomes of an outcomes managed approach to patients requiring prolonged ventilation. AJCC 1998;7:45–57.
30. Burns SM, Earven S. Improving outcomes for mechanically ventilated medical intensive care patients using advanced practice nurses: a six-year experience. Crit Care Nurs Clin North Am 2002;14:231–43.
31. Burns SM, Earven D, Fisher C, et al. Implementation of an institutional program to improve clinical and financial outcomes of patients requiring mechanical ventilation: one year outcomes and lessons learned. Crit Care Med 2003;31:2752–63.
32. Kress JP, Gehlbach B, Lacy M, et al. The long-term psychological effects of daily sedative interruption on critically ill patients. Am J Respir Crit Care Med 2003;168: 1457–61.
33. Ely EW, Inouye SK, Bernard GR, et al. Delirium in mechanically ventilated patients: validity and reliability of the confusion assessment method for the intensive care unit (CAM-ICU). JAMA 2001;286:2703–10.
34. Dubois MJ, Bergeron N, Dumaont M, et al. Delirium in an intensive care unit: a study of risk factors. Intensive Care Med 2001;27:1297–304.
35. Ely EW, Gautam S, Margolin R, et al. The impact of delirium in the intensive care unit on hospital length of stay. Intensive Care Med 2001;27:1892–900.
36. Ely EW, Shintani A, Truman B, et al. Delirium as a predictor of mortality in mechanically ventilated patients in the intensive care unit. JAMA 2004;291:1753–62.
37. Pandharipande PP, Shintani A, Peterson J, et al. Lorazepam is an independent risk factor for transitioning to delirium in intensive care unit patients. Anesthesiology 2006;104:21–6.
38. Burns SM. Adherence to sedation withdrawal protocols and guidelines in ventilated patients. Clin Nurse Spec 2012;26:22–8.
39. Elliott R, McKinley S, Aitken LM, et al. The effect of an algorithm-based sedation guideline on the duration of mechanical ventilation in an Australian intensive care unit. Intensive Care Med 2006;32:1506–14.
40. Williams TA, Martin S, Leslie G, et al. Duration of mechanical ventilation in an adult intensive care unit after introduction of sedation and pain scales. Am J Crit Care 2008;17:349–56.
41. Bucknall TK, Manias E, Presneill JJ. A randomized trial of protocol-directed sedation management of mechanical ventilation in an Australian intensive care unit. Crit Care Med 2008;36:1444–50.
42. MacIntyre NR, Cook DJ, Ely EW, et al. Evidence-based guidelines for weaning and discontinuing ventilatory support: a collective task force facilitated by the American College of Chest Physicians; the American Association for Respiratory Care; and the American College of Critical Care Medicine. Chest 2001;120(6 Suppl):375–95S.

43. Burns SM, Fisher C, Tribble S, et al. Multifactor clinical score and outcome of mechanical ventilation weaning trials: Burns Wean Assessment Program. Am J Crit Care 2010;19;431–40.

44. Burns SM, Fisher C, Tribble S, et al. The relationship of 26 clinical factors to weaning outcome. Am J Crit Care Nurs 2012;21:52–9.

45. Gawande A. The Checklist. The New Yorker Dec 10, 2007. Available at: http://www.newyorker.com/magazine/letters/2008/01/21/080121mama_mail4. Accessed September 30, 2011.

46. Brook AD, Sherman G, Malen J, et al. Early versus late tracheostomy in patients who require prolonged mechanical ventilation. Am J Crit Care 2000;9(5):352–9.

47. Freeman BD, Borecki IB, Coopersmith CM, et al. Relationship between tracheostomy timing and duration of mechanical ventilation in critically ill patients. Crit Care Med 2005;33(11):2513–20.

48. Nieszkowska A, Combes A, Luyt CE, et al. Impact of tracheotomy on sedative administration, sedation level, and comfort of mechanically ventilated intensive care unit patients. Crit Care Med 2005;33(11):2527–33.

49. Rumbak MJ, Newton M, Truncale T, et al. A prospective, randomized study comparing early percutaneous dilational tracheotomy to prolonged translaryngeal intubation (delayed tracheotomy) in critically ill medical patients. Crit Care Med 2004;32:1689–94.

50. Smyrnios NA, Connolly A, Wilson MM, et al. Effects of a multifaceted, multidisciplinary, hospital-wide quality improvement program on weaning from mechanical ventilation. Crit Care Med 2002;30:1224–30.

51. Burtin C, Robbeets C, Ferdinande P, et al. Early exercise in critically ill patients enhances short-term recovery. Crit Care Med 2009;37:2499–505.

52. Morris PE, Goad A, Thompson C, et al. Early intensive care unit mobility therapy in the treatment of acute respiratory failure. Crit Care Med 2008;36:2238–43.

53. Schweickert WD, Pohlman MC, Pohlman AS, et al. Early physical and occupational therapy in mechanically ventilated, critically ill patients: a randomised controlled trial. Lancet 2009;30:1824–6.

54. Thomsen GE, Snow GL, Rodriquez L, et al. Patients with respiratory failure increase ambulation after transfer to an intensive care unit where early activity is a priority. Crit Care Med 2008;36:1119–24.

55. Strom T, Martinussen T, Toft P. A protocol of no sedation for critically ill patients receiving mechanical ventilation: a randomised trial. Lancet 2010;6:475–80.

56. Thille AW, Harrois A, Schortgen F, et al. Outcomes of extubation failure in medical intensive care unit patients. Crit Care Med 2011;39:2612–8.

Self/Unplanned Extubation
Safety, Surveillance, and Monitoring of the Mechanically Ventilated Patient

Julie N. King, RN, MS, ACNP*, Valerie A. Elliott, MSN, ACNP

KEYWORDS

- Self/unplanned extubation • Risk assessment tool • Sedation • Restraints
- Quality improvement • Reintubation

KEY POINTS

- Risk factors for unplanned extubation include altered level of consciousness, use of analgesia and sedation medications, use of physical restraints, increased nursing workload, delirium, inadequate endotracheal tube fixation, and delayed ventilator weaning.
- Aggressive management of anxiety, agitation, pain, and delirium has the potential to decrease the risk of unplanned extubation.
- Physical restraints have not been shown to be effective at prevention of unplanned extubation; however, lower nurse-to-patient ratios and quality improvement programs for data tracking and staff education are recommended.
- The majority of patients who experience unplanned extubation do not require reintubation, suggesting current practices in weaning from mechanical ventilation are inadequate.
- Patients requiring reintubation have increased mortality and length of stay due to frequent complications.

For some must watch, while some must sleep.
                    William Shakespeare, "Hamlet"

The goals of health care professionals seem simple; provide quality care while preserving patient safety and well-being. For this goal to be possible, corrective and preventive measures to assure patient safety must be developed; in other words, protecting the patient against possible injury and negative outcomes.

Problems associated with mechanical ventilation (ie, ventilator-induced lung injury, barotrauma, volutrauma, atelectrauma, biotrauma, oxygen toxicity, and

Disclosures: Funding sources: none. Conflict of interest: none.
Weinberg Intensive Care Unit, Johns Hopkins Hospital, 401 North Broadway: Wbg 3A, Baltimore, MD 21231, USA
* Corresponding author.
E-mail address: jking47@jhmi.edu

ventilator-associated pneumonia) have been well-studied. Achieving the goal of maintaining airway patency and assuring adequate oxygenation and ventilation is sometimes disrupted, resulting in one of the least desirable outcomes, premature loss of airway due to unplanned extubation (UE).

UE is a serious concern to health care providers in the intensive care unit (ICU). UE is defined as a premature removal of the endotracheal tube (ETT)[1] by action of the patient (deliberate/self-extubation) or inadvertently during nursing care and manipulation of the patient.[2] UE is an event often considered to be an indicator of quality of care of mechanically ventilated patients.[3] UE often leads to adverse effects such as tracheal/laryngeal spasm or injury, inducing pulmonary or cardiac failure.[4]

The incidence of UE is reported to vary from .1 to 3.6 events per 100 events per 100 intubation days.[5] Of the UEs studied, deliberate self-extubations per 100 intubation days accounted for the majority of unplanned extubations, occurring at a rate of 50 to 100 unplanned extubations per 100 ventilated patients.[5] In one study, inadvertent/accidental UEs accounted for approximately 10% (range 3%–6%) of the cases.[6] Of these UEs, 60% of the cases required reintubation.[3,7]

There are numerous factors that have been shown to contribute to UE (self or inadvertent) including the location and cultures of the hospital. In a review of studies in the 1990s, UE was reported to be dependent on factors such as nursing care, timing of restraints, patient's level of consciousness, use of sedation, distribution of nursing labor, working hours, the physical setup of the ventilator, and delayed extubation.[8] A separate study of UEs in 122 patients showed that 55% of the patients were conscious, 68% of the patients were restrained. 46% of the patients required reintubation, and 7.3% of the patients incurred adverse effects, such as difficulties in intubation and tracheal spasm after UE.[4] An extensive review was performed of international and local studies. In a study of 139 patients in southern Taiwan, many factors were found to result in increased risk for UE such as gender, age, types of illness, duration of intubation, level of consciousness at extubation, anatomic route of intubation (oral greater than nasotracheal), use of restraints, and use of sedatives.[3] This study also identified a rate of UE at 6.4%. It was recommended that the medical provider and nurse should fully evaluate a patient's oxygenation status, decrease the length of the weaning for possible extubation, and remove the ETT promptly when extubation criteria are met.[3] Additionally, patients who are in the process of being weaned from the ventilator are more likely to sustain UE. Of noted importance, multiple investigators documented that UE was associated with prolonged duration of mechanical ventilation, ICU stay, and hospital stay compared with patients not having experienced UE.[3,7,9,10]

PATIENT EXPERIENCES DURING MECHANICAL VENTILATION

Currently, it is not always possible to determine which patients will experience a UE. Patients have multiple reasons to experience anxiety during mechanical ventilation. They are likely dealing with the knowledge of life-threatening illness and prognosis, or they may be recovering from a postsurgical procedure with an uncertain outcome. A significant relationship has been shown between the inability to communicate and feeling panic, insecurity, pain, and disturbances of sleep-wake cycles.[11] Their mobility is limited by the ventilator and attachment of monitors and invasive tubes/lines. The use of physical restraints may be necessary to assure patient safety, but certainly may be additive to their level of stress and anxiety.

A study of 150 patients who were mechanically ventilated for less than 48 hours in an adult ICU[12] showed that 50 (33%) did not remember being in an ICU or the ETT, 97 remembered being in the ICU, and 75 remembered the ETT. Sixty six percent of the patients who recalled the presence of an ETT reported being bothered moderately to extremely. More than half of those who remembered the ETT were bothered moderately to extremely by not being able to speak (68%), ETT discomfort (56%), and anxiety regarding the ETT (59%).

MONITORING OF CRITICALLY ILL PATIENTS

The ICU environment is dynamic and infused with sophisticated technology. It takes a skilled practitioner to appropriately recognize and properly diagnosis a problem. Understanding of the patient's past and current medical history along with an airway assessment are essential to proper decision-making. Not only are the providers responsible for being properly trained to monitor the mechanically ventilated patient, but they must also be experts on the traditional methods of assessment (inspection, palpation, percussion, and auscultation). Familiarity with equipment along with interpretation of laboratory data and changes in vital signs are essential skills. The primary goal of monitoring the mechanically ventilated patient is early detection of problems to prevent complications.

In the ICU, ventilated patients have several invasive lines and tubes, which assist in monitoring. Recognizing subtle changes in blood pressure, heart rate, cardiac rhythm, oxygen saturation, end tidal CO_2, urinary output, patient spontaneous respirations, and ventilator rate/pattern may help prevent an emergent situation. Also a basic check of the ventilator should be performed by trained personnel on a routine basis (usually the respiratory care practitioner). However, the care and safety of patients on ventilators are not one person's sole responsibility on the multidisciplinary ICU team. The ventilator should be checked to assure accurate settings as prescribed by the provider. Any irregularities should be corrected and brought to the attention of the appropriate person. All connections should be secured, and all alarms should be activated with appropriate alarm limits set.

When a patient seems in distress or anxious with increased work of breathing, a directed physical assessment may provide insight into the underlying cause. It is important to note and compare with previous assessments the type of artificial airway and position of the tube, skin color, temperature, moisture, crepitus, changes in breath sounds, and type and amount of secretions. Arterial blood gas analysis to monitor acid-base balance, as well as mixed venous and central venous saturation are more advanced methods of monitoring oxygen delivery and extraction. These are all required skills of the bedside nurse, respiratory therapist, and providers in the ICU to assist in the prevention of unplanned or accidental self-extubation.

PREVENTION OF UNPLANNED EXTUBATION
Patient Screening for Risk Factors

Given the numerous risk factors that can lead to UE, it is vital to develop a screening tool for mechanically ventilated patients to identify patients who are at increased risk. Early identification and treatment of modifiable factors may potentially lead to decreased incidence of UE and subsequently enhance quality of care.

A risk assessment tool (**Fig. 1**), called the Self-Extubation Risk Assessment Tool (SERAT) developed based on Bloomsbury Sedation Score and Glasgow Coma Scale (GCS) has been shown to have100% sensitivity and negative predictive values and 79% specificity.[13] This tool was therefore very good at identifying patients at risk for UE. However, it also had a high number of false-positives, which could lead to invasive therapies for patients who screened positive and might not necessarily go on to have UE. The SERAT tool in combination with early screening for factors noted by

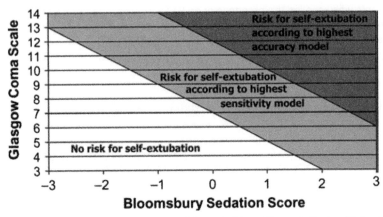

Fig. 1. Self Extubation Risk Assessment Tool (SERAT). (*From* Moons P, Boriau M, Ferdinande P. Self-extubation risk assessment tool: predictive validity in a real-life setting. Nurs Crit Care 2008;13(6):310–4; with permission.)

Fang and colleagues[8] could possibly be used in future research to develop a tool with both negative and positive predictive abilities.

Analgesia and Sedation

ICU patients typically have physical discomfort and anxiety related to multiple sources including disease physiology, invasive procedures, monitoring or therapeutic devices, nursing and respiratory care procedures, as well as prolonged immobility. Uncontrolled pain and anxiety have many negative effects on quality of care, including increased agitation and incidence of UE.[14] The goals of analgesia and sedation must be clearly established for each patient to ensure consistency among caregivers.

Current analgesia guidelines from the American College of Critical Care Medicine are summarized as follows[14]:

- Pain and response to analgesic therapies should be assessed via patient reporting on a numeric rating scale (0–10). For patients who cannot communicate, a subjective behavioral/physiologic rating tool should be used.
- Nonpharmacologic analgesic strategies (including heat/cold, massage, optimal positioning, and elimination of unnecessary devices, alarms, lights, noises, and so forth) should be used whenever possible to supplement pharmacologic analgesia such as including acetaminophen, nonsteroidal antiinflammatory drugs (NSAIDs), and opioids.
- Scheduled medication doses or a continuous infusion are preferable to "as-needed" dosing to ensure consistent analgesia.
- A patient who has the capacity to understand and operate a patient-controlled analgesia device will likely experience good quality of analgesia, less sedation, and less opioid consumption.
- NSAIDs or acetaminophen may be used as adjuncts to reduce overall opioid requirements.

Agitation and anxiety are commonly experienced by the patient requiring mechanical ventilation, affecting up to 50% to 74% of patients.[15,16] Agitation has been found to be a characteristic of patients with UE.[1,2,17,18] Frequent sources of anxiety in critically ill patients are related to an inability to communicate, lack of control, emotional distress regarding medical condition, unfamiliar noises and personnel, excessive stimulation, inadequate analgesia, frequent medical and nursing interventions, lack of mobility, and sleep deprivation. Administration of anxiolytics and sedating medications such as benzodiazepines, propofol (Diprivan), and dexmedetomidine (Precedex) are effective in relieving symptoms of anxiety and agitation.[14] Avoiding oversedation should be made a priority because it has been associated with prolonged mechanical ventilatory support, increased ICU length of stay, increased incidence of nosocomial infections, increased need for diagnostic testing, and overall increase in health care costs.[19] The practice of using intermittent, as-needed, boluses of sedation is a common factor in UE, and it has been shown that sedation and analgesia administered via continuous infusion may prevent UE in intubated patients who are alert.[20]

Nurse-driven sedation protocols based on frequent use of validated assessment tools such as the Ramsay Scale, Riker Sedation-Agitation Scale, Motor Activity Assessment Scale, and so forth, improve patient outcomes by reducing oversedation, duration of ventilator support, ventilator-associated pneumonia, and ICU length of stay.[19,21] Powers[22] showed that the use of a sedation protocol based on the Ramsay Scale significantly reduced UE.

Delirium: Screening and Treatment

Delirium is defined as the disturbance/fluctuation of consciousness with inattention, accompanied by acute changes in cognition over a short period of time.[23] There are many environmental and physiologic factors that predispose ICU patients to developing delirium. Recognition of factors such as advanced age, alcohol, tobacco and other drug use/history, hypertension, respiratory disease, preexisting cognitive impairment, depression, sensory impairment, restraints, catheters, psychoactive medications, sleep deprivation, hypoxemia, dehydration, hypotension, anemia, and renal or hepatic insufficiency are of importance in the prevention of delirium.[23] Regular screening of patients for hyperactive and hypoactive delirium is recommended, using a validated assessment tool such as the Confusion Assessment Method for ICU.[23]

The treatment of delirium starts with environmental considerations: reorientation to reduce confusion and agitation, encouraging normal sleep-wake cycles, avoidance of prolonged restraint use, and minimizing doses of sedatives or analgesics.[24] The presence of familiar persons such as family and friends is not protective against delirium[25]; however, comfort from an individual who is familiar with a patient's preexisting sources of stress and anxiety may decrease the incidence of psychosis in postoperative patients.[26]

Incidence and severity of symptoms of delirium are increased by inappropriate sedation and analgesia drug regimens. Sedatives are ineffective in the treatment of delirium, and patients will likely become more obtunded, confused, or agitated with their use.[14] The current Society of Critical Care Medicine guidelines for treatment of delirium in ICU patients describe neuroleptic agents such as haloperidol (Haldol) and chlorpromazine (Thorazine) as effective. This class of medication antagonizes dopamine-mediated neurotransmission at cerebral synapses and basal ganglia, causing a stabilizing effect on cerebral function.[14] Other medications identified as alternatives for treatment of delirium are atypical antipsychotics such as olanzapine (Zyprexa), risperidone (Risperdal), and quetiapine (Seroquel). These medications, however, have not been shown to be as effective as neuroleptics.[14]

Surveillance by Health Care Providers

Higher patient acuity and increased nurse/patient ratio have been shown to negatively affect many indicators of quality of care such as nosocomial infections, falls, medication errors, postoperative complications and UEs.[27] Increased vigilance by ICU staff has been shown to contribute to a decreased incidence of UE.[28,29] Also examined has been the level of nursing experience at time of UE. Patients in the care of more experienced ICU nurses (>4 years of experience) were found to have a lower rate of UE: 2.6%.[5,30] Many studies have reported that the optimal nurse/patient ratio for prevention of UE is 1:1.[31–33] Implementing this ratio universally in all mechanically ventilated patients may not be feasible from a financial standpoint; however, resources should be allocated to those patients who have been identified as at increased risk for UE.

Physical Restraints

Physical restraints are commonly used by health care providers to facilitate tolerance of medical care devices that cause discomfort and prevent premature or inadvertent removal of such devices. In recent times, ethical debates have critiqued use of physical restraints on patients without consent. It is important to limit the use of these devices to clinically appropriate situations, and only when alternative measures to reduce the patient's anxiety or agitation have failed.[34] For nearly 20 years, studies have shown that physical restraints are not effective at preventing UE.[24,35–39] Patients who are physically restrained have been shown to have a higher rate of unplanned extubation than those who are not restrained. A likely explanation for this finding is that staff applied the restraints in response to increased agitation or lack of cooperation with treatment/monitoring devices. Restraints have been shown to increase agitation,[1,40] thus increasing rates of UE. Determined patients have the ability to self-extubate even when they are restrained.[41] In contrast, Tominaga and colleagues[33] found an increase in the rates of unplanned extubation when their facility implemented a new policy strictly limiting the use of restraints. This result is consistent with the findings of Pesiri[42] that restraints can be useful in decreasing the number of UE. In other countries, overall rates of physical restraints usage is lower, with a greater focus on the appropriate use of sedation, early ventilator weaning, and secure fixation of the ETT than in the United States.[43]

ETT Fixation

Inadequate or insecure endotracheal fixation/securement leads to increased tube movement and discomfort, thus increasing the risk of UE.[4,5,17] With any ETT fixation method, health care providers must remain vigilant in maintaining the integrity of the oral mucosa and facial skin in order to prevent injury from excess/prolonged pressure on any given area. Commonly used methods for ETT fixation include commercial tube holder devices, various types of tape (cloth, plastic, paper, and so forth), circumferential versus face-only taping, and suturing or wiring the ETT to teeth/surrounding tissues; however, no single method has been demonstrated as superior.[44] It has been shown that ensuring proper attention and consistency in the method of securing the ETT decreases UE.[45] Standardizing a fixation method of both the ETT and ventilator tubing as a quality improvement program results in decrease in UE.[32,46]

Avoiding Prolonged Unnecessary Mechanical Ventilation

It has been widely established that the use of mechanical ventilation weaning protocols improves quality of care in critically ill patients by reducing overall duration of mechanical ventilation, incidences of UE, reintubation rates, and nosocomial infections such as ventilator-associated pneumonia.[1,20,29,32,41,46,47] Reintubation rates for patients who experience UE vary greatly depending on patient population, unit culture, and protocols, from 10.3%[48] to 78%,[24] with reduced duration of mechanical ventilation and shorter length of stay for those patients who do not require reintubation. These data suggest that a number of patients were ready to be weaned and possibly extubated but were not recognized as such by the health care team.

A widely accepted strategic approach to weaning has not yet been established, but is very much needed. A recent randomized controlled trial showed that standardized daily awakening trials (interruption of sedation medications with continuation of analgesia) in combination with spontaneous breathing trials are associated with a shorter duration of ventilation and ICU and hospital length of stay.[49] This study also demonstrated a significant reduction (32%) in 1-year mortality. Although this method of weaning remains somewhat controversial, it is likely that it will decrease UE and enhance quality of care for patients undergoing mechanical ventilation.[6]

Quality Improvement: Tracking/Reporting and Staff Education

Systematic reduction of adverse events such as UE is an important priority in improving the quality and safety of care for critically ill patients receiving mechanical ventilation. The European Society of Intensive Care Medicine recently formed a task force with the specific goal of improving the safety and quality of care provided to critically ill patients. This group came to a consensus on several quality of care indicators that will be used to drive future performance improvement initiatives. Decreasing the rate of UE is among the identified areas to be improved.[50] Considerable interest has grown in developing guidelines, protocols, bundles, checklists, and so forth, with the intent to reduce clinical variation, promote best practices, and improve outcomes.

Reporting of events to enable comparison of outcomes data across various health care facilities will assist in the identification of systematic problems leading to decreased quality of care. Focusing educational opportunities for health care staff aimed at these problems will likely improve patient outcomes related to UE and other outcomes. Focusing on quality improvement and safety promotes and encourages reporting of incidents instead of focusing on blame. Multiple investigators describe quality improvement initiatives involving patient screening, staff education, resource allotment, use of physical restraints, and protocols for sedation, analgesia, and weaning. Such initiatives show a reduction in UEs of 50% or more.[32,41,51,52]

MANAGEMENT OF UE

The sudden loss of an ETT leading to abrupt cessation of mechanical ventilation is associated with complications such as arrhythmias, hypotension, hypoxemia, emesis/aspiration, laryngeal trauma, respiratory distress/arrest, pneumonia, and atelectasis.[36,40,53,54] Approximately 31% to 78% will require reintubation after a UE due to inability to clear pulmonary secretions and meet ventilation/oxygenation demands.[53,55] These patients have increased mortality rates,[1,41,55] as well as higher rates of in-hospital complications and up to two times longer hospital length of stay.[24]

A conservative approach and initial supportive care are favorable when addressing UE. Providing supplemental oxygen, bronchodilators, assistance with clearing secretions, and elevating the head of bed may assist in alleviating initial distress. Automatic reintubation has not been shown to improve outcomes and should be avoided, particularly in situations where patients are being actively weaned from mechanical ventilation.[2] Patients undergoing weaning may tolerate UE and will experience the benefits of shorter length of stay and decreased risk of nosocomial infections.[36] Noninvasive pressure support ventilation may be an effective alternative to reintubation for up to 83% of patients with hypercarbic respiratory failure after extubation, because these patients showed improved gas exchange after 1 hour of therapy.[56]

The need to reestablish mechanical ventilator support will vary depending on the clinical situation. Patient characteristics and factors associated with a higher likelihood of requiring reintubation to restore mechanical ventilation are as follows:

- Decreased mental status related to sedation or illness (GCS <11) and impaired oxygenation (Pao$_2$/F io$_2$ <200).[1]
- Selected diagnosis, for example acute respiratory distress syndrome, chronic obstructive pulmonary disease, and pneumonia.[36]
- Chronic respiratory failure and increased ventilator-delivered minute ventilation.[17]
- Organ dysfunctions, infection, increase in pulmonary secretions, tachycardia, temperature greater than 37.5, pH greater than 7.45, poor pulmonary compliance, and nonpostoperative patient population.[28]

Immediate action is required when the need is to reestablish mechanical ventilation after a UE. A high incidence of difficult reintubations (up to 20%) and potential for airway loss can occur.[40,55] Frequent complications associated with reintubation after UE are multiple attempts at reintubation resulting in airway edema/trauma, inappropriate endotracheal tube placement, hypoxemia, bronchospasm, hypotension, arrhythmias, cardiac arrest, increased intracranial pressure, and need for a surgical airway.[57] Given the increased likelihood of difficult reintubation coupled with potential for life-threatening complications, it is critical that highly skilled personnel with advanced airway training be immediately available in the event of a UE.

SUMMARY

UE is a common problem in ICUs and is associated with prolonged duration of mechanical ventilation and ICU stay, thus posing a risk to safety and quality of patient care.

Primary prevention via risk screening is fundamental to the prevention of UE. Adequate analgesia and sedation, management of delirium, increased staff surveillance, judicious use of restraints, standardized tube fixation, aggressive weaning, and quality improvement initiatives are all known strategies to assist in decreasing UE. Given that many patients are likely to tolerate UE with supportive care, reintubation should not be considered mandatory. However, patients who require reintubation have increased mortality due to severe complications such as hypoxemia, bronchospasm, hypotension, arrhythmias, cardiac arrest, increased intracranial pressure, and need for surgical airway. Future research is needed to further develop standardized screening tools, sedation, analgesia, and delirium management protocols to decrease the incidence of UE and improve safety and quality of care.

REFERENCES

1. Chevron V, Menard JF, Richard J, et al. Unplanned extubation: risk factor of development and predictive criteria for reintubation. Crit Care Med 1998;26:1049–53.
2. Betbese AJ, Perez M, Bak E, et al. A prospective study of unplanned endotracheal extubation in intensive care unit patients. Crit Care Med 1998;26:1180–6.
3. Huang YT. Factors leading to self extubation of endotracheal tubes in the intensive care unit. Nurs Crit Care 2009;14:68–74.

4. Grap MJ, Glass C, Lindamond MO. Factors related to unplanned extubation of endotracheal tubes. Crit Care Nurse 1995;15:57–65.
5. da Silva PS, Fonseca MC. Unplanned endotracheal extubations in the intensive care unit: systematic review, critical appraisal, and evidence-based recommendations. Anesth Analg 2012;114(5):1003–14.
6. Bouza C, Garcia E, Diaz M, et al. Unplanned extubation in orally intubated medical patients in the intensive care unit: a prospective cohort study. Heart Lung 2007;36: 270–6.
7. de Lassence A, Alberti C, Azoulay E, et al. Impact of unplanned extubation and reintubation after weaning on nosocomial pneumonia risk in the intensive care unit: a prospective multicenter study. Anesthesiology 2002;97:148–56.
8. Fang L, Fang SH, Fang L. Results and clinical application-unplanned removal of endotracheal tube. J Med Sci 1999;28:328–31.
9. Krisnsey JS, Barone JE. The drive to survive: unplanned extubation in the ICU. Chest 2005;128:560–6.
10. Scott PH, Eigen H, Moye LA, et al. Predictability and consequences of spontaneous extubation in a pediatric ICU. Crit Care Med 1985;13:228–32.
11. Pierce L. Complications of mechanical ventilation and troubleshooting the patient ventilator system. In: Pierce L, editor. Management of the mechanically ventilated patient. St Louis (MO): Saunders Elsevier; 1995. p. 288–330.
12. Rontondi AJ, Chelluri L, Sirio C, et al. Patients recollections of stressful experiences while receiving prolonged mechanical ventilation in an intensive care unit. Crit Care Med 2002;30:746–52
13. Moons P, Boriau M, Ferdinande P. Self-extubation risk assessment tool: predictive validity in a real-life setting. Nurs Crit Care 2008;13(6):310–4.
14. Jacobi J, Fraser GL, Coursin DB, et al. Clinical practice guidelines for sustained use of sedatives and analgesics in the critically ill adult. Crit Care Med 2002;30(1):119–41.
15. Treggiari-Venzi M, Borgeat A, Fuchs-Buder T, et al. Overnight sedation with midazolam or propofol in the ICU: effects on sleep quality, anxiety and depression. Intensive Care Med 1996;22(11):1186–90.
16. Fraser G. Monitoring sedation, agitation, analgesia, and delirium in critically ill adult patients. Crit Care Clin 2001;17(4):1–16.
17. Boulain T. Unplanned extubations in the adult intensive care unit: a prospective multicenter study. Am J Respir Crit Care Med 1998;157:1131–7.
18. Woods JC, Mion LC, Connor JT, et al. Severe agitation among ventilated medical intensive care unit patients: frequency, characteristics and outcomes. Intensive Care Med 2004;30(6):1066–72.
19. Arnold HM, Hollands JM, Skrupky LP, et al. Optimizing sustained use of sedation in mechanically ventilated patients: focus on safety. Curr Drug Saf 2010;5(1):6–12.
20. Balon JA. Common factors of spontaneous self-extubation in a critical care setting. Int J Trauma Nurs 2001;7(3):93–9.
21. Popernack ML, Thomas NJ, Lucking SE. Decreasing unplanned extubations: utilization of the Penn State Children's Hospital Sedation Algorithm. Pediatr Crit Care Med 2004;5(1):58–62.
22. Powers J. A sedation protocol for preventing patient self-extubation. Dimens Crit Care Nurs 1999;18(2):30–4.
23. Morandi A, Jackson JC, Ely EW. Delirium in the intensive care unit. Int Rev Psychiatry 2009;21(1):43–58.
24. Atkins PM, Mion LC, Mendelson W, et al. Characteristics and outcomes of patients who self-extubate from ventilatory support: a case-control study. Chest 1997;112(5): 1317–23.

25. Dubois MJ, Bergeron N, Dumont M, et al. Delirium in an intensive care unit: a study of risk factors. Intensive Care Med 2001;27(8):1297–304.
26. Lazarus H, Hagens J. Prevention of psychosis following open-heart surgery. Am J Psychiatry 1968;124(9):1190–5.
27. Ream RS, Mackey K, Leet T, et al. Association of nursing workload and unplanned extubations in a pediatric intensive care unit. Pediatr Crit Care Med 2007;8(4):366–71.
28. Listello D, Sessler CN. Unplanned extubation. Clinical predictors for clinical extubation for reintubation. Chest 1994;105:1496–503.
29. Tindol GA Jr, DiBenedetto RJ, Kosciuk L. Unplanned extubations. Chest 1994;105(6):1804–7.
30. Yeh SH, Lee LN, Ho TH, et al. Implications of nursing care in the occurrence and consequences of unplanned extubation in adult intensive care units. Int J Nurs Stud 2004;41(3):255–62.
31. Marcin JP, Rutan E, Rapetti PM, et al. Nurse staffing and unplanned extubation in the pediatric intensive care unit. Pediatr Crit Care Med 2005;6(3):254–7.
32. Chiang A, Lee KC, Lee JC, et al. Effectiveness of a continuous quality improvement program aiming to reduce unplanned extubation: a prospective study. Intensive Care Med 1996;22(11):1269–71.
33. Tominaga GT, Rudzwick H, Scannell G, et al. Decreasing unplanned extubations in the surgical intensive care unit. Am J Surg 1995;170(6):586–9.
34. Maccioli GA, Dorman T, Brown BR, et al. Clinical practice guidelines for the mainte-nance of patient physical safety in the intensive care unit: use of restraining therapies–American College of Critical Care Medicine Task Force 2001–2002. Crit Care Med 2003;31(11):2665–76.
35. Curry K, Cobbs S, Kutash, M, et al. Characteristics associated with unplanned extubations in a surgical intensive care unit. Am J Crit Care 2008;17:45–51.
36. Whelan J, Simpson SQ, Levy H. Unplanned extubation. Predictors of successful termination of mechanical ventilatory support. Chest 1994;105(6):1808–12.
37. Chang LY, Wang KW, Chao YF. Influence of physical restraint on unplanned extuba-tion of adult intensive care patients: a case-control study. Am J Crit Care 2008;17(5):408–15.
38. Frezza EE, Carleton GL, Valenziano CP. A quality improvement and risk management initiative for surgical ICU patients: a study of the effects of physical restraints and sedation on the incidence of self-extubation. Am J Med Qual 2000;15(5):221–5.
39. Tung A, Tadimeti L, Caruna-Monaldo B, et al. The relationship of sedation to deliberate self-extubation. J Clin Anesth 2001;13:24–9.
40. Vassal T, Anh NG, Gabillet JM, et al. Prospective evaluation of self-extubations in a medical intensive care unit. Intensive Care Med 1993;19(6):340–2.
41. Maguire GP, DeLorenzo LJ, Moggio RA. Unplanned extubation in the intensive care unit: a quality-of-care concern. Crit Care Nurs Q 1994;17(3):40–7.
42. Pesiri AJ. Two year study of the prevention of unintentional extubation. Crit Care Nurs Q 1994;17(3):35–9.
43. Kapadia F. Unplanned extubation in medical and surgical ICUs. Intensive Care Med 2004;30(12):2289.
44. Gardner A, Hughes D, Cook R, et al. Best practice in stabilisation of oral endotracheal tubes: a systematic review. Aust Crit Care 2005;18(4):158:160–5.
45. Richmond A, Jarog D, Hanson V. Unplanned extubation in adult critical care: quality improvement and education payoff. Crit Care Nurse 2004;24:32–7.

46. Kollef M, Shapiro S, Silver P, et al. A randomized, controlled trial of protocol-directed versus physician-directed weaning from mechanical ventilation. Crit Care Med 1997; 25(4):567–74.

47. Ely E, Inouye S, Bernard G, et al. Delirium in mechanically ventilated patients. JAMA 2001;286(21):2703–10.

48. Jarachovic M, Mason M, Kerber K, et al. The role of standardized protocols in unplanned extubations in a medical intensive care unit. Am J Crit Care 2011;20(4): 304–11.

49. Girard TD, Kress JP, Fuchs BD, et al. Efficacy and safety of a paired sedation and ventilator weaning protocol for mechanically ventilated patients in intensive care (Awakening and Breathing Controlled trial): a randomised controlled trial. Lancet 2008;371(9607):126–34.

50. Rhodes A, Moreno RP, Azoulay E, et al. Prospectively defined indicators to improve the safety and quality of care for critically ill patients: a report from the Task Force on Safety and Quality of the European Society of Intensive Care Medicine (ESICM). Intensive Care Med 2012:598–605.

51. Sadowski R, Dechert RE, Bandy KP, et al. Continuous quality improvement: reducing unplanned extubations in a pediatric intensive care unit. Pediatrics 2004;114(3):628–32.

52. Birkett KM, Southerland KA, Leslie GD. Reporting unplanned extubation. Intensive Crit Care Nurs 2005;21(2):65–75.

53. Coppolo DP, May JJ. Self-extubations. A 12-month experience. Chest 1990;98(1): 165–9.

54. Bhattacharya P, Chakraborty A. Comparison of outcome of self-extubation and accidental extubation in ICU. Indian J Crit Care Med 2007;7(4):105–8.

55. Christie JM, Dethlefsen M, Cane RD. Unplanned endotracheal extubation in the intensive care unit. J Clin Anesth 1996;8(4):289–93.

56. Wysocki M, Tric L, Wolff M, et al. Noninvasive pressure support ventilation in patients with acute respiratory failure. Chest 1993;103(3):907–13.

57. Mort TC. Unplanned tracheal extubation outside the operating room: a quality improvement audit of hemodynamic and tracheal airway complications associated with emergency tracheal reintubation. Anesth Analg 1998;86(6):1171–6.

Early Mobilization in the Management of Critical Illness

Amy J. Pawlik, PT, DPT, CCS[a,b,*]

KEYWORDS

- Early mobilization • Critical care • Physical therapy • Occupational therapy
- Intensive care unit

KEY POINTS

- Critically ill and mechanically ventilated patients are at risk of developing neuromuscular and neurocognitive impairments.
- Mobilizing patients early in the course of critical illness may improve outcomes.
- Recent literature on early mobilization is reviewed, suggestions for implementation are discussed, and areas for future research are identified.

INTRODUCTION

Advances in medical care of critically ill patients have increased survival. However, patients who survive can be left with neuromuscular[1] and neurocognitive[2] impairments leading to impaired physical function[3–5] and decreased quality of life (QOL).[3,4,6,7] Recent attention has been directed toward the practice of pairing daily sedative interruption with physical activity very early in the course of medical management of patients who are mechanically ventilated and critically ill. Early mobilization has been shown to be feasible and safe,[8–10] decrease days on mechanical ventilation (MV),[11] decrease hospital and intensive care unit (ICU) lengths of stay,[9] and improve cognitive and functional outcomes.[11] Despite the research supporting early mobilization as an intervention to consider in the management of patients with critical illness, it can be challenging to implement and unanswered questions about its use and delivery remain. The standard of care regarding early mobilization and physical therapy involvement for patients in the ICU is highly varied depending on factors such as the type of facility (ie, academic vs community hospital)

The author has nothing to disclose.

[a] Therapy Services, University of Chicago Medical Center, MC 1081, W109, 5841 South Maryland Avenue, Chicago, IL 60637-1470, USA; [b] Cardiac and Pulmonary Rehabilitation, University of Chicago Medical Center, MC 1081, W109, 5841 South Maryland Avenue, Chicago, IL 60637-1470, USA
* Therapy Services, MC 1081, W109, 5841 South Maryland Avenue, Chicago, IL 60637-1470.
E-mail address: amy.pawlik@uchospitals.edu

Crit Care Nurs Clin N Am 24 (2012) 481–490
http://dx.doi.org/10.1016/j.ccell.2012.05.003
0899-5885/12/$ – see front matter © 2012 Published by Elsevier Inc.
ccnursing.theclinics.com

and the patient's clinical scenario (ie, cerebrovascular accident vs chronic obstructive pulmonary disease).[12] The purpose of this article is to review the current research addressing early mobilization in patients undergoing critical illness, discuss how it can be implemented into practice, and identify areas for future research.

IMMOBILITY AND DELIRIUM IN THE ICU

Management of critically ill patients has traditionally involved periods of immobility and bedrest and use of analgesic and sedative medications, and can require the use of MV. The deleterious effects of bedrest and medical management of critical illness have been well described.[13–16] Effects of bedrest are both physical and cognitive, including the presence of ICU-acquired weakness (ICU-AW)[14,15] and delirium.[16] Furthermore, deficits can develop rapidly. Skeletal muscle strength has been shown to decrease by 1% to 1.5% per day of bedrest.[17] In patients on MV, marked atrophy of diaphragmatic myofibers has been noted after 18 to 69 hours of inactivity and MV.[18] In patients who develop delirium during the first 5 days of ICU stay, nearly half (45.2%) develop delirium on the second day after ICU admission.[19]

Strength deficits after critical illness can be profound and impact both short- and long-term patient outcomes. The incidence of ICU-AW in patients mechanically ventilated for at least 7 days is 25% to 58%.[20,21] In patients awake enough to participate in the Medical Research Council Scale for Muscle Strength (MRC) assessment, 25% had ICU-acquired paresis.[20] In a study including nonresponsive patients with myopathy (established using electrophysiologic studies), the incidence of neuromuscular dysfunction was 58%.[21] Other studies have found this number to be even higher, between 50% and 100%.[22–24] The presence of neuromuscular dysfunction can contribute to difficulty weaning from the ventilator[25] and may be a predictor of prolonged ventilation.[26,27] In addition, the presence of ICU-AW has been associated with increased mortality.[21,28]

Studies suggest that cognitive function and physical function influence each other.[29] Delirium associated with critical illness (ie, ICU-acquired delirium) impacts a majority of patients who are mechanically ventilated.[2,30] It is characterized by changes in arousal and other cognitive deficits that can fluctuate and can occur early in the course of critical illness.[31] It requires the use of standard assessment measures, such as the Confusion Assessment Method for the ICU (CAM-ICU) for accurate identification.[32,33] Recently it has been noted that even validated tools such as the CAM-ICU may be suboptimal for identifying the presence of ICU delirium,[34] as sensitivity can be as low as 47%.[35] ICU-acquired delirium is independently associated with mortality.[2,36] Risk of death at 6 months[2] and 1 year[36] has been shown to increase 10% for every day spent with delirium. The presence of ICU-acquired delirium is also associated with longer hospital stay[30,37] and increased ICU and hospital costs.[38]

The impact of critical illness is not limited to a patient's ICU stay. The physical and cognitive impairments can persist long after hospital discharge, having profound effects on a patient's physical function and QOL. Survivors of acute respiratory distress syndrome (ARDS) demonstrate persistent weakness 1 year after critical illness, and only 50% of ICU survivors are able to return to work.[3] Patients demonstrate ambulation distance on the 6-minute walk test[39] that is reduced from norms 1[3,5] and 2 years[5] after critical illness and have reduced QOL at 12[6] and 23 months[7] after discharge from the hospital and ICU, respectively. These deficits persist even when pulmonary function returns to near normal.[3] Herridge and colleagues[4] found that, in ARDS survivors, exercise capacity and mean score on the physical component of the Medical Outcomes Study 36-Item Short-Form Health

Survey (SF-36)[40] were below normative values even 5 years after discharge from the ICU, despite return of pulmonary function to normal.[4] In addition, lack of early mobility in the ICU has been associated with increased hospital readmission and death.[41]

Risk factors for the debilitating deficits associated with critical illness are many. Factors contributing to ICU-AW include systemic inflammation, seen as a response to sepsis and multisystem organ dysfunction. In addition, the use of medications such as corticosteroids and neuromuscular blocking agents, abnormal blood glucose levels, and immobility can contribute to ICU-AW.[1] Hypoglycemia and immobility can also contribute to neurocognitive changes, along with hypotension, hypoxemia, and sedation.[42] Research aimed at controlling the multiple medical factors that may contribute to weakness and delirium is ongoing. Addressing immobility has been a recent "hot topic" toward which many groups are focusing in an effort to improve overall patient outcomes.

CAUSES OF IMMOBILITY IN THE ICU

Immobility in the ICU is related to a number of factors. One is the use of sedative and analgesic drugs for critically ill patients undergoing MV. Drugs such as benzodiazapines, propofol, haloperidol, and opiates are often initiated to manage agitation and anxiety and facilitate medical care.[43] Addressing the effect of sedative use on patient outcomes, Kress and colleagues[44] described findings from a trial in which daily sedative interruption was performed, allowing patients to be awake and able to follow commands. This intervention was shown to be feasible and safe and resulted in a reduction in duration on MV and a reduction in ICU length of stay (LOS).[44]

To build upon this intervention, a controlled trial paired periods of sedation interruption with physical therapy (PT) and occupational therapy (OT) very early in the patient's hospital course.[11] PT and OT sessions were coordinated with daily interruption of sedation. Therapy sessions consisted of assisting the patient to sit at the edge of the bed, stand, ambulate, and perform activities of daily living such as dressing and grooming, even in the presence of MV and an endotracheal tube. Patients in the intervention group received PT and OT on average 1.5 days after intubation.[11] The majority of sessions (68%) were conducted while subjects were intubated and on MV.[8] Patients who received early PT and OT demonstrated significant return to independent functional status (59% vs 35% of patients, $P = .02$) as measured by the Functional Independence Measure (FIM),[45] increased ambulation distance (33.4 vs 0 m, $P = .004$) at time of hospital discharge, more ventilator-free days (23.5 vs 21.1, $P = .05$), and 50% fewer days of delirium (2 vs 4, $P = .02$) at time of hospital discharge. Those in the control group received PT and OT 7.4 days after intubation.

Other studies have shown that mobilizing patients who are mechanically ventilated via an endotracheal tube is feasible and safe[46,47] and that patients mobilized early in their ICU stay have decreased ICU and hospital LOS.[9] In addition to the practice of facilitating out of bed activity (eg, sitting, standing, and walking), use of cycle ergometry, in which the legs are cycled actively or passively as the patient remains in bed,[48] and electrical muscle stimulation[49,50] have shown promising results. Finally, protocols and algorithms have been described to help with decision making regarding initiation and progression of early mobilization and exercise.[9,51,52]

WHAT IS READY FOR IMPLEMENTATION INTO PRACTICE?

As with many medical practices, there are questions regarding early mobilization that warrant further exploration. However, there are some relative certainties. To implement an

Table 1	
Care process model	
Stage	Description of Activity
1	Establish sense of urgency.
2	Create a powerful guiding coalition (including unit nurse manager, physician director, and others).
3	Create a vision (priority goals were identified).
4	Communicate the vision.
5	Empower others to act on the vision.
6	Plan for and create short-term wins (change data was provided to staff).
7	Consolidate improvements and produce more change.
8	Institutionalize new approaches.

Adapted from Hopkins RO, Spuhler VJ, Thomsen GE. Transforming ICU culture to facilitate early mobility. Crit Care Clin 2007;23(1):81–96; with permission.

early mobilization program, one must first have practitioners in a variety of disciplines who support the effort to mobilize patients early. Second, the coordination of care among a variety of critical care specialists must be addressed. Finally, there must be processes in place to facilitate the creation of an individualized plan for each patient to ensure timely and successful early mobilization.

It is clear that the approach to implementing early mobilization involves the entire care team. Gaining support from team members can be difficult, as there may be a perception that changing practice in the ICU may add a great deal of time and effort[53] to an already busy workload. The culture of an ICU may or may not endorse mobilizing patients who have traditionally been kept on bedrest. Reasons for this include insufficient knowledge of clinical outcomes, tendency to resist change, and the fact that ICU practitioners are often removed from the difficulties patients can face at the time of hospital discharge.[53] However, a number of groups have addressed the issue of culture as a hindrance to change.[10,54]

Hopkins and colleagues[54] described the creation of an ICU, dedicated to improving outcomes for patients who were physiologically stable but still required MV. Mobilization was made a key priority and the article comprehensively describes the steps taken (**Table 1**) to ensure cooperation from all staff members. Among other initiatives, outcome data were collected and shared with the staff on a regular basis to reinforce the culture of early mobility. Positive outcomes included increased ambulation distance, with 69% of patients having ambulated more than 100 feet on the last day of treatment in the ICU and decreased ICU and hospital LOS by 3 days and 4 days respectively.[47] In another project, a full-time PTs and OTs were dedicated to the ICU as part of a larger quality improvement project designed to increase the utilization of therapy services. Needham and colleagues[10] describes a 4-month quality improvement project in which processes were implemented to create an environment conducive to early mobilization. Changes included the modification of standard activity orders on medical ICU (MICU) admission to read "as tolerated" and a change in sedation practices that encouraged the use of "as needed" bolus doses rather than continuous intravenous infusions. Guidelines for seeking consultation with a PT or OT were developed; a PT, OT, and rehabilitation assistant were added to the MICU staff, and referrals to physiatry and neurology increased. In addition, significant education on complications of critical illness, benefits of early activity, sedation practice, and training related to rehabilitation of patients on MV was provided to all involved practitioners. Compared to the period of time before the initiation of the new processes, more patients received PT and/or OT while in the MICU (70% vs 93%, $P = .04$), patients received more rehabilitation sessions per patient (1 vs 7, $P<.001$) and demonstrated improved outcomes including improved sedation and delirium status (MICU days alert [30% vs 67%, $P<.001$] and not delirious [21% vs 53%, $P = .003$]).[10]

Mobilization in the ICU requires coordination of care. For example, to successfully mobilize a patient who is mechanically ventilated, sedation must be withheld, the patient must be assessed for level of arousal and presence or absence of delirium, ventilatory needs must be assessed (with ventilator settings altered as needed), and coordination with therapists must occur for the patient to be seen during periods of sedation interruption. Completing these steps traditionally would require bedside nurses and physicians who are responsible for assessing level of arousal and presence or absence of delirium, managing sedation, and, with the addition of respiratory therapists, implementing spontaneous breathing trials. Each step traditionally requires a designated health care professional to recognize when his or her contribution is required and to intervene accordingly.

Rather than maintain the practice whereby each practitioner focuses only on his or her typical responsibilities, a setting in which there is collaboration and overlap of duties (within their scope of practice) can better promote practices that improve patient outcomes. An example of this was outlined by Hopkins and colleagues when describing the creation of their specialty ICU. They describe a culture in which the roles of the members of the ICU team overlap and that additional training is provided so, for example, a nurse can initiate a respiratory treatment if the respiratory therapist is busy ambulating a patient.[54]

Once the team has been established, creating a standardized series of objectives may be of benefit. A suggested example of this was developed by Vasilevskis and colleagues.[29] The authors describe an approach to managing the patient undergoing MV by which evidence-based therapies are "bundled" together in an effort to improve outcomes. Their "bundle," abbreviated ABCDE, acknowledges that the optimal management of the intubated patient does not consist of early mobility alone but of multiple factors that need to be addressed. Along with mobilization, patients undergo sedative interruption, spontaneous breathing trials, and monitoring of delirium and level of sedation. It is a potentially useful outline of the steps needed to optimize the care of the patient who is critically ill and undergoing MV. The components of the bundle and an associated interdisciplinary model for its execution are outlined in **Table 2**, suggesting that the initiation of each of the components may become the responsibility of all professional disciplines, even requiring a change in the unit's traditional scope of practice.

Admittedly, the suggestions in **Table 2** and the example of a dedicated mobility unit[54] require individuals motivated to champion the implementation of a new process, an adequate number of staff and those proficient in treating patients undergoing critical illness, and, often, support from hospital administration. In some institutions, creating a formalized program in which support is given from all those who impact the hospital culture (administration, physicians, nurses, therapists, etc.) can be daunting and prevent the initiation of any implementation of early mobilization if "buy in" is not achieved at all levels. In these instances, it may be more feasible to approach a change in practice one patient at a time, working toward the aforementioned culture change in a gradual fashion, rather than trying to make global system changes at one time.

Table 2		
Components of ABCDE bundle and suggested facilitators of each component		
Component	Facilitated by	Frequency

A Awake
Daily interruption of sedation (DIS)
  or spontaneous awakening trials
  (SATs)
	Physicians
	Nurse practitioners
	Bedside nurses
	Physical and occupational therapists
		Daily

B Breathing trial Spontaneous breathing trial (SBT)	Physicians Nurse practitioners Bedside nurses Respiratory therapists	Daily
C Choice of sedation and novel sedation regimens	Physicians Nurse practitioners	Daily
D Delirium monitoring and treatment	Physicians Nurse practitioners Bedside nurses Physical and occupational therapists	Daily
E Early mobility and exercise	Physical and occupational therapists Bedside nurses Respiratory therapists	Daily

Data from Vasilevskis EE, Ely EW, Speroff T, et al. Reducing iatrogenic risks: ICU-acquired delirium and weakness-crossing the quality chasm. Chest 2010;138(5):1224–33.

AREAS FOR FUTURE STUDY

Although the data supporting early mobilization are promising, questions remain as ICU culture and practice evolve. These include staffing, ensuring safety regarding mobilization in the presence of medical devices and support, and extending the body of literature to include long-term outcomes.

A concern that frequently arises in the discussion of early mobility is the potential impact on care provider staffing. Some of the challenges are staffing (shortage of nurses and physical and occupational therapists). Other challenges relate to the realities of costs, that is, the attention paid to optimizing health care dollars spent per patient. Therefore, it is necessary to address the impact of early mobilization on overall hospital cost and the availability and feasibility of adding staff in ICUs. The first question is whether additional staff is required. In the study by Morris and colleagues,[9] utilization of therapy services was much higher in the intervention group. In addition, more than 50% of patients in the usual care group did not receive therapy services at any point during hospital admission. Conversely, in the randomized controlled trial (RCT) published by Schweickert and colleagues,[11] patients in the control group versus the intervention group participated in a similar duration of therapy, once they were extubated, and 95% of patients in the control group received therapy but received it later in the hospital stay. These data suggest that patients who have been in the ICU are receiving therapy; it is just occurring at varying points of time in the hospital course. The implications for staffing remain unclear and will require further study. In assessing the potential financial implications of early mobilization, there was not a difference in hospital costs per patient in the protocol versus the group receiving the usual care despite the presence of a dedicated ICU mobility team.[9]

The optimal team of practitioners required to perform early mobilization safely, effectively, and efficiently has yet to be determined. Studies have described two,[8] three,[9,10] and four[54] practitioners being present to mobilize patients undergoing MV, with the team including variations of groups of practitioners including nurses, respiratory therapists, PTs, OTs, and nursing and therapy technicians. Differences in outcomes between each combination of practitioners have not been described. Differences have been noted in the level of mobility achieved when mobilization was performed by nurses versus PTs.[55] PTs achieved more advanced levels of mobility but nurses and PTs described different reasons for deferring mobility. For example, nurses rated hemodynamic instability (26% vs 12%, $P = .03$) and renal replacement therapy (12% vs 1%, $P = .03$) more highly as barriers whereas PTs identified neurologic impairment as a higher-rated barrier (18% vs 38%, $P = .002$). More study is needed to determine the optimal team to perform mobility and perhaps make the process more standardized from one institution to the next.

Additional study is also required to determine when patients with certain medical devices and support are safe for mobilization. It is often a common practice that patients with femoral vascular access devices are placed on bedrest.[56] There is little published research to support or refute this practice. A case series of 30 subjects in 47 physical therapy sessions[56] recently found no complications with the mobilization of patients with femoral arterial catheters, providing some support for this practice. However, additional study is needed and the investigation of mobilization with other femoral devices such as those used for hemodialysis would be useful. Another issue regarding the medical management of critically ill patients is mobilization when medications are used to enhance hemodynamic stability. A published early mobilization algorithm suggests that activity should be initiated in the absence of catecholamine drips.[52] Conversely, Pohlman and colleagues[8] described the mobilization of patients on two or more vasoactive drugs, and other studies have deferred activity if vasoactive requirements have recently increased[9,10] but the presence of the drug alone did not preclude activity. Another possible complication is the use of continuous renal replacement therapy (CRRT). As CRRT can be in use during much of a 24-hour period, it has the potential to derail a mobility plan if activity is not performed while the therapy is in use. It has been shown[8] that it is possible to mobilize patients while they are receiving CRRT, provided the site of access is not femoral. In this author's experience, it is possible to safely mobilize a patient with femoral dialysis access when the device is not in use and, in some cases, even when the device is in use. This requires further study and, ideally, the use of superior access sites[57] (whenever possible) may allow mobilization of the patient to occur.

Finally, it is yet unclear what the long-term implications of early mobilization may be. Controlled studies investigating early mobilization[9,11] describe outcomes only to the time of hospital discharge. Further study is needed to determine whether early mobilization produces lasting benefits that positively impact functional status and QOL after discharge.

SUMMARY

The use of MV to help manage critical illness is projected to increase steadily in the coming years.[58] Patients undergoing MV cannot afford to wait until extubation to engage and participate in activity. Studies have shown that the use of early mobilization can prevent some of the negative sequelae of critical illness and ongoing studies aim to further describe the safety and benefit of this intervention and to direct clinicians in changing practice in their own institutions.

REFERENCES

1. Schweickert WD, Hall J. ICU-acquired weakness. Chest 2007;131(5):1541–9.

2. Ely EW, Shintani A, Truman B, et al. Delirium as a predictor of mortality in mechanically ventilated patients in the intensive care unit. JAMA 2004;291(14):1753–62.

3. Herridge MS, Cheung AM, Tansey CM, et al. One-year outcomes in survivors of the acute respiratory distress syndrome. N Engl J Med 2003;348:683–93.

4. Herridge MS, Tansey CM, et al. Functional disability 5 years after acute respiratory distress syndrome. N Engl J Med 2011;364:1293–304.

5. Cooper AB, Ferguson ND, Hanly PJ. Long-term follow-up of survivors of acute lung injury: lack of effect of a ventilation strategy to prevent barotrauma. Crit Care Med 1999;27(12):2616–21.

6. Davidson TA, Caldwell ES, Curtis JR, et al. Reduced quality of life in survivors of acute respiratory distress syndrome compared with critically ill control patients. JAMA 1999; 281(4):354–60.

7. Angus DC, Musthafa AA, Clermont G, et al. Quality-adjusted survival in the first year after the acute respiratory distress syndrome. Am J Respir Crit Care Med 2001;163: 1389–94.

8. Pohlman MC, Schweickert WD, Pohlman AS, et al. Feasibility of physical and occupational therapy beginning from initiation of mechanical ventilation. Crit Care Med 2010;38:2089–94.

9. Morris PE, Goad A, Thompson C, et al. Early intensive care unit mobility therapy in the treatment of acute respiratory failure. Crit Care Med 2008;36:2238–43.

10. Needham DM, Korupolu R, Zanni JM, et al. Early physical medicine and rehabilitation for patients with acute respiratory failure: a quality improvement project. Arch Phys Med Rehabil 2010;91:536–42.

11. Schweickert WD, Pohlman MC, Pohlman AS, et al. Early physical and occupational therapy in mechanically ventilated, critically ill patients: a randomised controlled trial. Lancet 2009; 373:1874–82.

12. Hodgin KE, Nordon-Craft A, McFann KK, et al. Physical therapy utilization in intensive care units: results from a national survey. Crit Care Med 2009;37(2):561–8.

13. Brower RG. Consequences of bed rest. Crit Care Med 2009;37(10 Suppl):S422–8.

14. Chambers MA, Moylan JS, Reid MB. Physical inactivity and muscle weakness in the critically ill. Crit Care Med 2009;37(10 Suppl):S337–46.

15. Stevens RD, Dowdy DW, Michaels RK, et al. Neuromuscular dysfunction acquired in critical illness: a systematic review. Intensive Care Med 2007;33(11):1876–91.

16. Ouimet S, Kavanagh BP, Gottfried SB, et al. Incidence, risk factors and consequences of ICU delirium. Intensive Care Med 2007;33(1):66–73.

17. Topp R, Ditmyer M, King D, et al. The effect of bed rest and potential of prehabilitation on patients in the intensive care unit. AACN Clin Issues 2002;13(2):263–76.

18. Levine S, Nguyen T, Taylor N, et al. Rapid disuse atrophy of diaphragm fibers in mechanically ventilated humans. N Engl J Med 2008;358(13):1327–35.

19. Lin S, Huang C, Liu C, et al. Risk factors of the development of early-onset delirium and the subsequent clinical outcome in mechanically ventilated patients. J Crit Care 2008;23(3):372–9.

20. De Jonghe B, Sharshar T, Lefaucheur JP, et al. Paresis acquired in the intensive care unit: a prospective multicenter study. JAMA 2002;288:2859–67.

21. Leijten FS, Harinck-de Weerd JE, Poortvliet DC, et al. The role of polyneuropathy in motor convalescence after prolonged mechanical ventilation. JAMA 1995;274(15): 1221–5.

22. Witt NJ, Zochodne DW, Bolton CF, et al. Peripheral nerve function in sepsis and multiple organ failure. Chest 1991;99:176–84.

23. Berek K, Margreiter J, Willeit J, et al. Polyneuropathies in critically ill patients: a prospective evaluation. Intensive Care Med 1996;22:849–55.

24. De Jonghe B, Cook D, Sharshar T, et al. Acquired neuromuscular disorders in critically ill patients: a systematic review: groupe de Reflexion et d'Etude sur les Neuromyopathies En Reanimation. Intensive Care Med 1998;24:1242–50.

25. Hund EF. Neuromuscular complications in the ICU: the spectrum of critical illness-related conditions causing muscular weakness and weaning failure. J Neurol Sci 1996; 136(1–2):10–6.

26. Garnacho-Montero J, Amaya-Villar R, Garcia-Garmendia JL, et al. Effect of critical illness polyneuropathy on the withdrawal from mechanical ventilation and the length of stay in septic patients. Crit Care Med 2005;33(2):349–54.

27. De Jonghe B, Bastuji-Garin S, Sharshar T, et al. Does ICU-acquired paresis lengthen weaning from mechanical ventilation? Intensive Care Med 2004;30(6):1117–21.

28. Garnacho-Montero J, Madrazo-Osuna J, Garcia-Garmendia JL, et al. Critical illness polyneuropathy: risk factors and clinical consequences. A cohort study in septic patients. Intensive Care Med 2001;(27)8:1288–96.

29. Vasilevskis EE, Ely EW, Speroff T, et al. Reducing iatrogenic risks: ICU-acquired delirium and weakness-crossing the quality chasm. Chest 2010;138(5):1224–33.

30. Ely EW, Gautam S, Margolin R, et al. The impact of delirium in the intensive care unit on hospital length of stay. Intensive Care Med 2001;27:1892–900.

31. American Psychiatric Association. Diagnostic and statistical manual of mental disorders. 4th edition. Washington, DC: American Psychiatric Press; 2000.

32. Spronk PE, Riekerk B, Hofhuis J, et al. Occurrence of delirium is severely underestimated in the ICU during daily care. Intensive Care Med 2009;35(7):1276–80.

33. van Eijk MM, van Marum RJ, Klijn IA, et al. Comparison of delirium assessment tools in a mixed intensive care unit. Crit Care Med 2009;37(6):1881–5.

34. Patel SB, Kress JP. Accurate identification of delirium in the ICU: problems with translating the evidence in the real-life setting. Am J Respir Crit Care Med 2011; 184(3):287–8.

35. van Eijk MM, van den Boogaard M, van Marum RJ, et al. Routine use of the confusion assessment method for the intensive care unit: a multicenter study. Am J Respir Crit Care Med 2011;184(3):340–4.

36. Pisani MA, Kong SY, Kasl SV, et al. Days of delirium are associated with 1-year mortality in an older intensive care unit population. Am J Respir Crit Care Med 2009;180(11):1092–7.

37. Thomason JW, Shintani A, Peterson JF, et al. Intensive care unit delirium is an independent predictor of longer hospital stay: a prospective analysis of 261 non-ventilated patients. Crit Care 2005;9(4):R375–81.

38. Milbrandt EB, Deppen S, Harrison PL, et al. Costs associated with delirium in mechanically ventilated patients. Crit Care Med 2004;32(4):955–62.

39. Butland RJ, Pang J, Gross ER, et al. Two-, six-, and 12-minute walking tests in respiratory disease. Br Med J (Clin Res Ed) 1982;284(6329):1607–8.

40. Ware JE Jr, Kosinski M, Gandek B. SF-36 health survey manual & interpretation guide. Lincoln, RI: Quality Metric; 2005.

41. Morris PE, Griffin L, Berry M, et al. Receiving early mobility during an intensive care unit admission is a predictor of improved outcomes in acute respiratory failure. Am J Med Sci 2011;341(5):373–7.

42. Desai SV, Law TJ, Needham DM. Long-term complications of critical care. Crit Care Med 2011;39(2):371–9.

43. Shelly MP. Sedation, where are we now? Intensive Care Med 1999;25:137–9.

44. Kress JP, Pohlman AS, O'Connor MF, et al. Daily interruption of sedative infusions in critically ill patients undergoing mechanical ventilation. N Engl J Med 2000;342: 1471–7.

45. Keith RA, Granger CV, Hamilton BB, et al. The functional independence measure: a new tool for rehabilitation. Adv Clin Rehabil 1987;1:6–18.
46. Thomsen GE, Snow GL, Rodriguez L, et al. Patients with respiratory failure increase ambulation after transfer to an intensive care unit where early activity is a priority. Crit Care Med 2008;36:1119–24.
47. Bailey P, Thomsen GE, Spuhler VJ, et al. Early activity is feasible and safe in respiratory failure patients. Crit Care Med 2007;35:139–45.
48. Burtin C, Clerckx B, Robbeets C, et al. Early exercise in critically ill patients enhances short-term functional recovery. Crit Care Med 2009;37:2499–505.
49. Gerovasili V, Stefanidis K, Vitzilaios K, et al. Electrical muscle stimulation preserves the muscle mass of critically ill patients: a randomized study. Crit Care 2009;13:R161.
50. Routsi C, Gerovasili V, Vasileiadis I, et al. Electrical muscle stimulation prevents critical illness polyneuromyopathy: a randomized parallel intervention trial. Crit Care 2010; 14:R74.
51. Gosselink R, Clerckx B, Robbeets C, et al. Physiotherapy in the intensive care unit. Neth J Crit Care 2011;15(2):66–75.
52. Hanekom S, Gosselink R, Dean E, et al. The development of a clinical management algorithm for early physical activity and mobilization of critically ill patients: synthesis of evidence and expert opinion and its translation into practice. Clin Rehabil 2011;25(9): 771–87.
53. Bailey PP, Miller RR 3rd, Clemmer TP. Culture of early mobility in mechanically ventilated patients. Crit Care Med 2009;37(10 Suppl):S429–35.
54. Hopkins RO, Spuhler VJ, Thomsen GE. Transforming ICU culture to facilitate early mobility. Crit Care Clin 2007;23(1):81–96.
55. Garzon-Serrano J, Ryan C, Waak K, et al. Early mobilization in critically ill patients: patients' mobilization level depends on health care provider's profession. PM R 2011;3(4):307–13.
56. Perme C, Lettvin C, Throckmorton TA, et al. Early mobility and walking for patients with femoral arterial catheters in intensive care unit: a case series. JACPT 2011;2(1): 30–4.
57. Raman J, Loor G, London M, et al. Subclavian artery access for ambulatory balloon pump insertion. Ann Thorac Surg 2010;90(3):1032–4.
58. Needham DM, Bronskill SE, Calinawan JR. Projected incidence of mechanical ventilation in Ontario to 2026: preparing for aging baby boomers. Crit Care Med 2005; 33(3):574–9.

Telemedicine in the Intensive Care Unit

Marilyn Nielsen, RN-BC, MS[a,*], Jodi Saracino, RN-BC, BSN[b]

KEYWORDS

- Tele-ICU • Critical care • Telemedicine • Nursing

KEY POINTS

- It is estimated if each hospital implemented intensivist physician staffing, approximately 55,000 lives and $4.3 billion dollars could be saved in the United States.
- Research suggests the quality of care in intensive care units (ICUs) varies, and better outcomes are achieved in ICUs staffed by intensivists versus an attending physician.
- However, there is a limited supply of new critical care specialists as teaching hospitals have decreased the size of critical care programs for financial reasons.
- Tele-ICU solutions have been recommended as a means to help support facilities who do not have or cannot maintain full time critical care medicine specialist coverage.

INTRODUCTION

Today hospitals face significant challenges owing to the need for health care reform. There are financial issues resulting from continuing national economic problems, an increased number of unemployed and uninsured patients, decreased number of admissions, and more denials for payment. It is proposed that hospitals will receive rewards if they can demonstrate quality outcomes and there will be a monetary penalty for facilities with high readmission rates and no payment for conditions that that were not present-on-admission. In critical care areas, the call for the needed focus on patient safety and outcomes and the need to provide evidence-based quality care is challenging not only because of existing economic issues, but also because of a growing critical care crisis.[1–3] Factors that the critical care crisis can be attributed to include a growing elderly population, shortage of intensivists, and lack of critical care nurses.

The authors have nothing to disclose.

[a] Clinical Informatics, Littleton Adventist Hospital, Centura Health System, 7700 South Broadway, Littleton, CO 80122, USA; [b] Clinical Informatics, Catholic Health Initiatives, 198 Inverness Drive West, Englewood, CO 80112, USA

* Corresponding author.

E-mail address: marilynnielsen@centura.org

Crit Care Nurs Clin N Am 24 (2012) 491–500
http://dx.doi.org/10.1016/j.ccell.2012.06.002
0899-5885/12/$ – see front matter © 2012 Elsevier Inc. All rights reserved.

As the U.S. population has been aging, the risk of mortality has been falling. In 1950, the total percentage of the U.S. population older than the age of 65 was approximately 8%; the percentage increased to 12.5% in 2009 and it is projected to be 20% by 2050.[4] In addition, the composition of the U.S. population is becoming more diverse. This is impacting health care needs and challenges health care planning because of differences between racial and ethnic groups and their access to health care services and health insurances.[4,5]

Approximately 500,000 intensive care unit (ICU) patients in the United States die each year. It is estimated if each hospital implemented intensivist physician staffing, approximately 55,000 lives and $4.3 billion dollars could be saved in the United States.[6,7] Research suggests the quality of care in ICUs varies and better outcomes are achieved in ICUs staffed by intensivists versus an attending physician.[7–9] However, there is a limited supply of new critical care specialists as teaching hospitals have decreased the size of critical care programs for financial reasons. It is predicted by 2020, there will be a 35% shortfall of intensivists and pulmonologists, and this will increase to 46% by 2030.[10]

The ongoing shortage in experienced nurses who specialize in intensive care is due to numerous factors. There is a shortage of nursing faculty, which limits nursing school enrollments. Fewer young adults are entering the nursing profession (ICUs historically attract younger nurses), and the current RN workforce is aging, with the average age around 44.5 years. Staffing on nursing units is insufficient, resulting in increased stress levels that lead to job dissatisfaction and nurses leaving the profession. Finally, it is taking 7% longer to staff a critical care vacancy.[11]

RECOMMENDATIONS TO IMPLEMENT TELE-ICU

Today there are government incentives for the implementation of a certified electronic health record (EHR). While the EHR is being emphasized as an avenue to improve health care by facilitating communication among providers, decreasing medical errors, and as a means to enhance clinical decision making, more solutions are needed to improve the health care system and help to ensure care is affordable and accessible. Telemedicine solutions need to be considered. These systems have the potential to equalize disparities in access, increase a health system's efficiency, and promote patient-centered care in local environments.[12]

The Leapfrog Group, a U.S. health advisory board of Fortune 500 companies, has identified key evidence-based recommendations to improve the quality of health care, decrease mortality, and overall reduce ICU costs.[6] This group has encouraged ICU physician staffing (IPS) as one of its safety standards because of the potential benefits for patients. Research has shown a 30% reduction in hospital mortality and a 40% reduction in ICU mortality in hospital ICUs where critical care specialists manage or co-manage all patients. Another recommendation from the Leapfrog group is the use of telemedicine (tele-ICU) to provide coverage in facilities that cannot support a full-time specialist in critical care medicine and as an adjunct to facilities without 24-hour intensivist coverage.[7,9,13]

TELE-ICU CARE MODEL

The tele-ICU care model consists of a team of critical care specialists (intensivists), experienced critical care nurses, and in some cases pharmacists, who are located in a remote central command center. Tele-ICUs typically provide 24/7 critical care nursing coverage, while intensivist coverage can vary from 24 hours a day to coverage provided only through the night. The tele-ICU team does not replace bedside patient care and should be viewed as an additional tool to help improve patient safety and outcomes.[13]

Specifically, tele-ICU personnel proactively engage in the care of the patient via:

- System hardware transmitting patient physiologic data via secure Web connections
- Display of device information (eg, IV pump settings and ventilator settings)
- Access to laboratory studies and radiographic images
- Access to nursing, respiratory therapy, and physician documentation
- Embedded decision support systems to track data and give alerts if a negative trend is occurring.[13,14]

Within a remote command center, each eICU RN sits at a workstation. A workstation typically contains two computers that have been configured to three or four display monitors each. A multiline telephone is available along with earpiece and microphone. There is a high-resolution remote camera that can be used to visually access a patient. A ringing bell within the patient's room might be used so bedside staff are aware when the camera has been activated. The eICU RN would then provide his or her name and state the purpose for turning on the camera.[15,16]

A basic principle of the tele-ICU is routine rounding and attention to evidence-based practices to help prevent complications. The eICU RN conducts rounds anywhere from every hour to every 4 hours depending on the acuity of the patient. During rounds, patient orders, the plan of care, laboratory results, radiology, and other tests are reviewed. The eICU RN then applies his or her critical care thinking skills to assess how the patient is doing. Throughout a shift, any alerts that appear on the computer screen would be addressed. An eICU system interfaces with bedside monitoring systems, and the decision support system built into eICU system can help to identify subtle changes and trends in the patient's laboratory studies and physiologic parameters (eg, vital signs, urine output). The alerts may be color coded based on severity. The eICU RN would then review the patient's data and hemodynamic information to troubleshoot the alert. If unable to determine the cause, the remote camera would be turned on to visualize the patient and ICU room to see if the bedside nurse is with the patient and aware of any alarms. If the alert is valid and the bedside RN is not aware, the eICU RN would phone appropriate bedside staff and could make suggestions for an assessment or intervention.[13,15,16]

When the ePhysican is on duty, she or he may only round on high-acuity patients or those patients who have deteriorating trends in vital signs. The ePhysician can read and interpret test results, provide consultation, and may write orders as indicated. Other duties for eICU staff might include assisting with new admissions, supervising procedures, responding to emergencies, or serving as a resource when called upon. Staff within an eICU command center work together as a team. They respect and support each and often depend on each other to help answer questions that might come from bedside staff.[15,16]

Robotic devices are a newer approach for a tele-ICU, and their use is growing as these devices can have lower equipment costs. The robot is about 6 feet tall and equipped with two cameras, a display monitor, and microphone. It uses an Internet connection and video conferencing for real-time two-way audio–video communications, along with robotic control software that allows multidirectional movement. Access is achieved via the hospital's secure intranet, or via an encrypted virtual private network.[17] The robot can move from one patient to the next. There is the ability to capture video images of the patient and to communicate directly with the bedside caregivers, the patient, and his or her family. The robot would not replace daily intensivist rounding. Use of such a device has an advantage of allowing many members of the multidisciplinary critical care team to observe rounds from a location outside of the patient's room such as a conference room. There can be limitations to these devices if there are wireless connectivity issues, and the range for obtaining video images is lower compared to that of wall-mounted cameras that can be utilized with a remote tele-ICU command center.[14,17]

BENEFITS OF A TELE-ICU

Remote intensivists and experienced critical care nurses can help identify subtle changes in a patient's condition through the use of decision support software and alerts and they can provide timely feedback to bedside staff. For example, further investigation into decreased oxygenation, hypotension, tachycardia, or abnormal laboratory results allows for early identification and initiation of goal-directed therapy for conditions such as sepsis or stroke symptoms.[18] The remote clinicians can also help with adherence to standard best practice guidelines, which can lead to fewer ventilator days and ventilator-acquired pneumonias and improve blood glucose management.[16] Early initiation of evidence-based practices can help to lower the number of ICU days, improve patient outcomes, and lower overall hospital costs.[14,19–22] There is also an advantage of having health care professionals available for immediate consultation if needed. Along with intervening on behalf of the patient, off-site staff can share information and provide reassurance and education to bedside staff.[14,23]

Many rural communities in the United States face not only a lack of trained critical care physicians but also a shortage of primary care physicians and nurses. Use of a tele-ICU has the potential to decrease health care inequalities in regions with limited or no specialists and to enhance the in-person care that is available.[23]

Although use of robotic devices is limited at this time, it is interesting to note that in one survey of family members and patients around the use of robots in an ICU the technology received positive reviews, and many felt it was beneficial to care and they supported continued use. There are other possible benefits of robotics in that noise and traffic in ICUs during rounding might be decreased, leading to improved patient and staff satisfaction.[17]

TELE-ICU CHALLENGES AND ISSUES

As of 2009, it was estimated there were 4900 adult ICU beds being supported by a tele-ICU program and more than 1 million patients had been monitored via a tele-ICU.[14] Although tele-ICU is promising and its use increasing over the past decade, it still has not been widely adopted because of multiple issues and challenges. These include cost, staff acceptance, privacy issues, and lack of face-to-face interaction with the provider and licensure.

The cost of installing a full tele-ICU command center and paying salaries for tele-ICU staff is reportedly approximately $6 to $8 million, and this is beyond the investment for an electronic medical record system. Once established, a tele-ICU command center can have annual operating costs around $1 to $2 million, which would include maintenance costs, any needed licenses, and staffing expenses. There may be additional needs to upgrade existing hardware or software systems of the physical ICU because they may not be compatible with the tele-ICU system. Many hospitals simply lack the needed financial resources to acquire and maintain a tele-ICU, and this remains a major barrier.[24]

Currently, there is limited or no patient/insurance billing and reimbursement for tele-ICU physician services. Costs for tele-ICU personnel need to be assumed by the hospital or health care system and may vary depending on the staffing model used in the command center.[14,25] In 2010, the Center for Medicare and Medicaid Services established a reimbursement telemedicine code, but it applies only to facilities that are not in large metropolitan areas. Reimbursement issues are a barrier for many facilities. It has been suggested that tele-ICU systems could be used for a limited number of beds in a facility, and only the sickest patients would be monitored. This could help reduce costs for installing and operating the full range of equipment; however, more studies are needed.[22,26]

While only 10% of U.S. hospitals utilize tele-ICU coverage, adoption by other facilities is likely. Studies assessing the impact of tele-ICU coverage on patients do not always look at the impact on ICU staff specifically. ICU staff must not only work with remote tele-ICU clinicians, but they have to implement and operate the system within their department. It has been noted that overall, physicians and nurses view tele-ICUs favorably; however, over the past decade there has not been a great deal of research. Many of the studies often lack methodologic rigor and there is a need for better evaluation of tele-ICU remote monitoring that addresses benefits, challenges, and workflow dynamics for ICU staff.[27–29]

For facilities looking at implementing a tele-ICU, some strategies have been identified that can help facilitate staff acceptance, such as:

- Include ICU clinicians in the design and implementation of a tele-ICU.
- Build support for tele-ICU coverage among ICU staff before rollout.
- Coordinate clinicians from the monitoring center and bedside teams to build trust on both sides of the camera.
- Audiovisual contact is better than audio contact alone.
- Hire ICU command center intensivists and critical care nurses who are skilled in interpersonal communication to reduce any perceived threat by bedside clinicians.[27,29,30]
- Designate an ICU champion who supports the new technology to help manage staff needs and decrease the stress accompanying the change.
- Allow time for sufficient training on the use of tele-ICU equipment.

Nurses have identified concerns around patient and family acceptance of tele-ICU, with some nurses having expressed worries that tele-ICU is intrusive to their daily workflow and decreases patient privacy. Issues of feeling "spied upon" have also been conveyed and concerns voiced that time at the bedside would be adversely impacted, as staff would have to deal with tele-ICU devices.[28]

Suggestions to help ease these concerns include having ICU staff meet and get to know remote telemedicine staff, as well as the requirement that there is two-way video conferencing available with the remote command center.[29] Also, policies should be established around the use of the in-room cameras, speakers, and microphones and that these devices be activated only upon request of the bedside staff when help is needed or during established rounds.[28]

When dealing with tele-ICUs, the patient cannot choose his or her remote caregiver, and probably will not have the opportunity to meet the responsible intensivist in the command center if he or she works off-hours or weekends. With critically ill patients, a decision may need to be made with no physician available on site to explain a complex treatment or have options explained to the patient or family members. This could place unwanted responsibility on nursing staff. Having video conferencing readily available could be used to help facilitate communications with off-site intensivists, but this can have limitations as well if a sensitive conversation needs to occur.[23]

Since 1998 and the development of a mutual recognition model of nursing licensure, nurses licensed in their home state can practice in other states under their respective state's Nurse Practice Act, if that state is part of the interstate compact. Currently 24 states have enacted the nurse licensure compact. Additional work continues toward reducing licensure barriers impacting tele-ICU nursing.[31]

OUTCOMES RESEARCH

In 2011, the American College of Chest Physicians recognized a lack of high-quality, peer-reviewed research on the value of tele-ICU for patients and hospital systems. To provide a conceptual and practical framework for tele-ICU research needs, a working group came together sponsored by the Critical Care Societies Collaborative. This group includes the American Association of Critical Care Nurses, the American College of Chest Physicians, the American Thoracic Society, and the Society of Critical Care Medicine. A research agenda was subsequently proposed to advance the science of tele-ICU as a strategy to improve the quality of health care.[32]

The working group noted that a tele-ICU research framework should include many clinical disciplines. In addition, two major components were identified to help standardize reporting across studies:

1. Assessment of the preimplementation ICU environment (baseline) and
2. A standardized language defining the tele-ICU interventions. This could include whether tele-ICU monitoring is continuous or intermittent, the training and composition of the remote team (eg, physicians, nurses, pharmacists), and the goal of the program.[32]

The working group recommended three interrelated research domains organized around the Donabedian framework for health care quality. The domains include the structure of tele-ICU programs, the process of tele-ICU medicine, and the effect of telemedicine on critical care outcomes.[32,33]

Research topics related to the structure of a tele-ICU program include looking at the makeup and core competencies of the tele-ICU team, determining the impact of tele-ICU on existing staffing patterns, and identifying teamwork and traditional communication patterns impacted within the ICU.[32]

Research topics related to the process of tele-ICU medicine include tele-ICU delivery how to measure and improve tele-ICU workflow, how communication influences whether tele-ICU recommendations are acted on by staff, and investigating how telemedicine can help improve adherence to evidence-based practices in the ICU.[32]

Proposed telemedicine outcomes research include investigating the effect of tele-ICU on patient mortality and quality of life, looking at the impact of tele-ICU on patient and family satisfaction, and the effects of telemedicine on length of stay or patient readmissions rates.[32]

The demand for accountable care is growing. Public and private purchasers of health benefits are looking for increased safety, quality, and cost-effective care for the people they cover, and performance scores on the quality of care a facility provides are to be publicly reported. It is important that along with this growth, the focus of research continues in the area of understanding the strengths of telemedicine. Future research areas should include how to best use telemedicine to improve the care, what outcomes are best achieved with telemedicine, and the cost effectiveness of remote ICU care.[2,32]

IMPLICATIONS FOR NURSING PRACTICE

A major step in recognizing tele-ICU nursing as a professional specialty came in April 2011, with the launch of the Association of Critical Care Nurses (AACN) CCRN-E certification. This certification is an extension of the traditional CCRN certification program and is the first credential designation of tele-ICU nursing.[34]

Tele-ICU nursing expands the role of the ICU nurse beyond the traditional role of hands-on at the bedside, by having nurses provide care and expertise at a distance, using state of the art technology. Working in the tele-ICU command center encourages autonomy, a sense of teamwork, and professional growth. Without this technology, small changes in a patient's condition might go undetected. This additional layer of care and second set of eyes on a patient can be especially beneficial for novice nurses. The knowledge and wisdom of the remote nurse can quickly be accessed via phone or audiovisual technology, thus providing a level of reassurance to bedside staff.[2,35]

Tele-ICU nurses must have significant experience and the ability to communicate effectively with a variety of personalities. Most have 5 to 15 years or more of experience in the ICU setting. Some are attracted to the tele-ICU because bedside nursing is physically and emotionally demanding. Others are attracted to this growing field because it is fast paced, challenging, and rewarding. Some tele-ICU nurses work at both the bedside and in a tele-ICU to maintain their clinical competence.[34]

Strategies for remote staff to demonstrate competency can be time consuming, as the command center may service many hospitals simultaneously. Most remote centers do not require competencies be completed for each hospital; instead there is a system-wide competency program. Estimates are a tele-ICU nurse can spend 2 to 10 hours on validation criteria and competency assessments.[34] For the tele-ICU nurse to positively impact patient outcomes and to be a leader in clinical change, it has been suggested that these nurses demonstrate the following:

- Strong perceptive and observational skills
- Skill with technology utilized in the remote command center
- Ability to work within a facility's clinical information system
- Ability to critically think and utilize knowledge from clinical experiences
- Ability to make independent decisions based on the situation
- Strong interpersonal and communication skills
- Willingness to work at a high level of collaboration with ICU clinicians.[2,34]

FUTURE DIRECTIONS

One area where telemedicine has demonstrated significant benefit, because of the emergent nature of the condition, is in stroke care. Tele-stroke programs are being implemented and have been instrumental in early diagnosis and intervention. These programs leverage the care of neurologic specialists using audio–video technology in areas where access to such specialized care may otherwise be out of reach, or many hours away. Medications to treat stroke must be given within a narrow window of time after the onset of symptoms so emergent diagnosis is essential. A telemedicine solution that reaches out to community and rural areas will aid in the early identification and intervention for these patients, resulting in better outcomes. The integration of tele-stroke programs continues to grow nationwide.[36]

Tele-ICUs are beginning to expand to areas outside of the ICU, such as the emergency department and post-anesthesia care, labor and delivery, and medical–surgical units. This extension to other areas where there are often patients with a high acuity level facilitates early communication with an intensivist and an eICU RN. In addition, the tele-ICU could be used during an epidemic or mass casualty situation to help network intensivists and trauma surgeons to on-site physicians. Use of robots outside of the ICU is also being investigated. The hope is a mobile unit could be deployed with rapid response team activations and code management teams, thus extending the expert support of the remote intensivist out to floor patients.[13,16]

As the use of remote care delivery systems grows, nurse educators are faced with challenges on how to best train and prepare students for a future where technologies such as robotics and tele-ICUs have a presence. These technologies in the health care environment require technical expertise, but there is also a need for training on how to effectively collaborate and communicate with remote clinicians to facilitate critical point-of-care decisions. Digital health care will continue to expand and nurses of the future need the skill set to work within this environment.

Nursing should continue to research and identify best practices on how to implement and incorporate evolving technologies, such as a tele-ICU, into the nurse's workflow at the bedside while keeping patient safety and care goals at the forefront.

Rapidly growing demands for highly skilled critical care staff and the aging U.S. population are increasing the need for the use of telemedicine programs in various areas of health care, including the ICU. Utilizing tele-ICU technology to aggregate resources stands to improve the quality of care, can help to lower hospital costs, and has the potential to improve patient outcomes.[2]

REFERENCES

1. Healthcare Information and Management Systems Society (HIMSS). Call to action enabling healthcare reform using information technology recommendations for the Obama administration and 111th Congress. Available at: http://www.himss.org/2009calltoaction/himsscalltoactiondec2008.pdf. Accesssed April 23, 2012.
2. Rufo R. Using the tele-ICU care delivery model to build organizational performance, part 1. Crit Care Nurs Q 2011;34(3):177–81.
3. Rufo R. Tele-ICUs, part 2: adding value to the health care equation. Crit Care Nurse Q 2011;34(3):182–6.
4. Shrestha LB, Heisler EJ. The changing demographic profile of the United States. Congressional Research Service. Available at: http://www.fas.org/sgp/crs/misc/RL32701.pdf. Accessed April 28, 2012.
5. Vincent GK, Velkoff VA. The next four decades the older population in the United States: 2010 to 2050. U.S. Census Bureau. Available at: http://www.census.gov/prod/2010pubs/p25-1138.pdf. Accessed April 28, 2012.
6. Lwin AK, Shepard DS. Estimating lives and dollars saved from universal adoption of the Leapfrog safety and quality standards: 2008 Update. Schnieder Institutes for Health Policy. Available at: http://www.leapfroggroup.org/media/file/Lives_Saved_Leapfrog_Report_20Final_(2).pdf. Accessed March 28, 2011.
7. Pronovost P, Angus DC, Dorman T, et al. Physician staffing patterns and clinical outcomes in critically ill patients: a systematic review. JAMA 2002;288(17):2151–62.
8. Nguyen YL, Kahn JM, Angus DC. Reorganizing adult critical care delivery: the role of regionalization, telemedicine, and community outreach. Am J Respir Crit Care Med 2010;181(11):1164–9.
9. Leapfrog. Fact sheet—ICU Physician Staffing (IPS). Available at:http://www.leapfroggroup.org/media/file/FactSheet_IPS.pdf. Accessed March 28, 2011.

10. Angus DC, Kelley MA, Schmitz RJ, et al. Caring for the critically ill patient. Current and projected workforce requirements for care of the critically ill and patients with pulmonary disease: can we meet the requirements of an aging population? JAMA 2000;284(21):2762–70.

11. American Association of Colleges and Nursing (AACN). Nursing shortage fact sheet. Available at: http://www.aacn.nche.edu/media-relations/NrsgShortageFS.pdf. Accessed April 14, 2012.

12. Bashshur R, Shannon GW. National telemedicine initiatives: essential to healthcare reform. Telemed J E Health 2009;15(6):600–10.

13. Jarrah S, Van der Kloot TE. Tele-ICU: remote critical care telemedicine. PCCSU July 1. 2010;24. Available at: http://www.chestnet.org/accp/pccsu/tele-icu-remote-critical-care-telemedicine?page=0,3. Accessed May 14, 2011.

14. Lilly CM, Thomas EJ. Tele-ICU: experience to date. J Intensive Care Med 2010;25(1): 16–22.

15. Stafford TB, Myers MA, Young A, et al. Working in an eICU unit: life in the box. Crit Care Nurs Clin North Am 2008;20(4):441–50.

16. Myers MA, Reed KD. The virtual ICU (vICU). Crit Care Nurs Clin North Am 2008;20(4): 439–9.

17. Sucher J, Todd S, Jones S, et al. Robotic telepresence: a helpful adjunct that is viewed favorably by critically ill surgical patients. Am J Surg 2011;202(6):843–7.

18. Loyola S, Wilhelm J, Fornos J. An innovative approach to meeting early goal-directed therapy using telemedicine. Crit Care Nurs Q 2011;34(3):187–99.

19. Lilly CM, Cody S, Zhao H, et al. Hospital mortality, length of stay and preventable complications among critically ill patients before and after tele-ICU reengineering of critical care processes. JAMA 2011;305(21):2175–83.

20. Breslow MJ, Rosenfeld BA, Doerfler M, et al. Effect of a multiple-site intensive care unittelemedicine program on clinical and economic outcomes: an alternative paradigm for intensiviststaffing. Crit Care Med 2004;32(1):31–8.

21. Willmitch B, Golembeski S, Kim SS, et al. Clinical outcomes aftertelemedicine intensive care unit implementation. Crit Care Med 2012;40(2):450–4.

22. Franzini L, Sail KR, Thomas EJ, et al. Costs and cost-effectiveness of a telemedicine intensive care unit program in 6 intensive care units in a large health care system. J Crit Care 2011;26(3):329, e321–6.

23. Nesher L, Jotkowitz A. Ethical issues in the development of tele-ICUs. J Med Ethics 2011;37(11):655–7.

24. New England Healthcare Institute. Massachusetts Technology Collaborative. Critical care, critical choices: the case for tele-ICUs in intensive care. Available at: http://www.nehi.net/publications/49/critical_care_critical_choices_the_case_for_teleicus_ in_intensive_care. Accessed May 20, 2012.

25. New England Healthcare Institute. Massachusetts Technology Collaborative. Tele-ICUs: remote management in intensive care units. Available at: http://www.nehi.net/ publications/13/teleicus_remote_management_in_intensive_care_units. Accessed May 20, 2012.

26. Rogove HJ, McArthur D, Demaerschalk BM, et al. Barriers to telemedicine: survey of current users in acute care units. Telemed J E Health 2012;18(1):48–53.

27. Young BL, Chan PS, Cram P. Staff acceptance of tele-ICU coverage: a systematic review. Chest 2011;139(2):279–88.

28. Shahpori R, Hebert M, Kushniruk A, et al. Telemedicine in the intensive care unit environment-a survey of the attitudes and perspectives of critical care clinicians. J Crit Care 2011;26(3):328, e9–15.

29. Mullen-Fortino M, DiMartino J, Entrikin L, et al. Bedside nurses' perceptions of intensive care unit telemedicine. Am J Crit Care 2012;21(1):24–3.

30. Goran SF. A second set of eyes: an introduction to tele-ICU. Crit Care Nurse 2010;30(4):46–55.

31. National Council of State Board of Nursing. Nurse Licensure Compact. Available at: https://http://www.ncsbn.org/nlc.htm. Accessed May 17, 2012.

32. Kahn JM, Hill SH, Lilly CM, et al. The research agenda in ICU telemedicine: a statement from the critical care societies collaborative. Chest 2011;140:230–8.

33. Donabedian A. The quality of care. How can it be assessed? JAMA 1988:260(12): 1743–8.

34. Goran SF. A new view: tele-intensive care unit competencies. Crit Care Nurse 2011;31(5):17–29.

35. Goran SF. Making the move: from bedside to camera-side. Crit Care Nurse 2012; 32(1):e20–9.

36. Schwamm LH, Audebert HJ, Amarenco P, et al. Recommendations for theimplementation of telemedicine within stroke systems of care: a policy statement from the American Heart Association. Stroke 2009;40:2635–60. Available at: http://stroke.ahajournals.org/content/40/7/2635.full.pdf+html. Accessed June 10, 2012.

Index

Note: Page numbers of article titles are in **boldface** type.

Crit Care Nurs Clin N Am 24 (2012) 501–508
http://dx.doi.org/10.1016/S0899-5885(12)00077-9
0899-5885/12/$ – see front matter © 2012 Elsevier Inc. All rights reserved.

Printed and bound by CPI Group (UK) Ltd, Croydon, CR0 4YY

03/10/2024

01040456-0013